Articular Cartilage Tribology
关节软骨摩擦学

李 锋 著

中国海洋大学出版社

·青岛·

图书在版编目（CIP）数据

关节软骨摩擦学:英文 / 李锋著 . -- 青岛:中国
海洋大学出版社，2020. 11
ISBN 978-7-5670-2638-4

Ⅰ. ①关… Ⅱ. ①李… Ⅲ. ①关节软骨－关节损伤－
诊疗－英文 Ⅳ. ① R681. 3

中国版本图书馆 CIP 数据核字（2020）第 224521 号

出版发行	中国海洋大学出版社			
社　　址	青岛市香港东路 23 号		邮政编码	266071
出 版 人	杨立敏			
网　　址	http://pub.ouc.edu.cn			
订购电话	0532－82032573（传真）			
责任编辑	邵成军		电　　话	0532－85902533
印　　制	日照日报印务中心			
版　　次	2020 年 11 月第 1 版			
印　　次	2020 年 11 月第 1 次印刷			
成品尺寸	170 mm ×240 mm			
印　　张	11. 25			
字　　数	201 千			
印　　数	1—1000			
定　　价	45. 00 元			

Preface

In 1973, the term of biotribology was introduced by Dowson, the professor of Leeds University. In the beginning, the main aim of this new research area is mainly to focus on friction and wear problems in the human body. The application can be an artificial organ related to the ailments and physiological changes. After several years, the domain of biotribology increased as more researchers participated in other areas. The research area of biotribology has extended to skin, tendon, ligament, artificial heart valve, genitals, and contraceptive equipment. The research content of biotribology includes almost all frictional problems in the biological system, and the research focus is the structure of the human body, illness, trauma, orthopedic surgery, and so on. In recent years, as the area is extending quickly, several new areas are contained. Moreover, the problems in biotribology have also become a typical scale problem. People study the macroscopic scale and micro-scale problems in this area. Biotribology is also a rapidly emerging and developing interdiscipline and it becomes a hot area in the engineering field and medical field that can relieve the pain of patients in the hospital.

This book aims at the friction and wear of articular cartilage and artificial joint materials. It uses various detection methods to compare and study the basic properties of human articular cartilage, bovine articular cartilage, and artificial cartilage. Most of the content in this book is adapted from the author's past related research papers and dissertations; due to time constraints, the positions in the original text are not marked.

This book was supported by Shandong Provincial Key Research and Development Program (SPKR & DP) (2017GGX30108) and Qingdao Original Innovation Program Basic Research for Application Project (17-1-1-92-jch).

Li Feng

College of Electromechanical Engineering

Qingdao University of Science and Technology

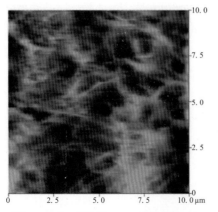

Figure 3-1   AFM Image of the Human
Cartilage Surface

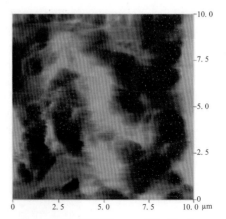

Figure 3-2   AFM Image of the Bovine
Cartilage Surface

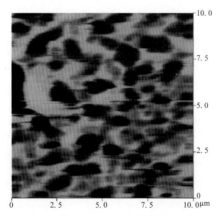

Figure 3-3   AFM Image of PVA Hydrogel Surface

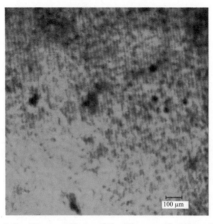

Figure 4-5   Contact State of the Human Cartilage Surface

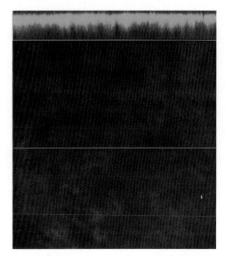

Figure 4-6   Slice Graph of Contact Area

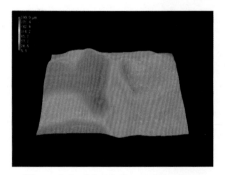

Figure 7-4   Morphology of Cartilage
Surface

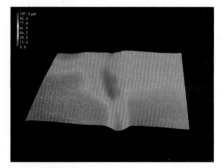

Figure 7-5   Morphology of Cartilage
Surface

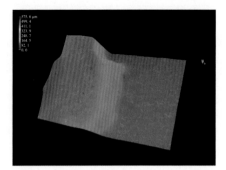

Figure 7-6   Morphology of Cartilage
Surface

Contents

Chapter 1
Articular Cartilage and Biotribology

1.1　Biomaterials and Biotribology

Biomaterials can be called biomedical materials, which are artificial materials. Biomaterials are used to replace the natural materials with synthetic materials in the living tissues in the human body. From the 1960s to the 1970s, the first generation of biomaterials emerged. Since then, different biomaterials had become a hot research topic in the world.

Biomaterials have been used in the medical field for a long time. Since the emerging of humankind, people have been fighting with different diseases. Biomaterials are a key tool to fight these diseases. In about 3500 BC, the ancient Egyptians used cotton fiber and horse mane as a suture line to suture wounds. The usage of cotton fiber and horse mane can be regarded as the earliest application of biomaterials in the human body. The Indians in Mexico had used timber to mend the human bone. In about 2500 BC, dental prosthesis, nasal prosthesis, and auricle prosthesis emerged in graves of China and Egypt. People had used golden plates to repair the patent's jawbone defection. The bone fracture related to metal fixator was recorded in the late 18th century. A lot of metal plates had been used as tools to fix the fracture of bones which was emerged in the 1800s. A dental implant made of gold appeared in 1809. In 1851, vulcanized natural rubber was processed into artificial denture and jawbone.

Organ failure and tissue defection are one of the most serious problems for human beings and account for more than 50% of medical expenses. In the early 20th century, the development of new high molecular material induced a systematic study of the artificial organ which started clinical application in 1940.

Since the usage of the artificial organ was developed, a lot of material that was not designed for medical use was applied in the clinical field. There are several common characteristics of various biological materials. They should be made into single equipment or implanted with some medicine. They can treat, enhance, or replace certain body tissues. But they cannot harm the body after implantation.

In the area of the cardiovascular implant, man-made vascular graft was woven from Nylon. However, the degradation of Nylon occurred and the implants were broken *in vivo*. Nylon was eliminated in the material selection of artificial implant aftermath. In recent years, Polyester (Dacron), polytetrafluoroethylene (PTFE), polyurethane (PU) and natural mulberry silk is chosen to woven man-made vascular graft and is applied to clinical in a large number of fields, for example, treatment of aortic fistula, aortic stricture, resection and replacement of superior and inferior vena cava. In November 2015, the researchers of Japan's national center for circulatory organ diseases declared that a man-made vascular graft with the diameter being as small as 0.6 mm was developed. This small man-made vascular graft was the world's smallest vascular graft and could be used in vascular bypass surgery of the human brain and heart.

After the First World War, the first generation of biological materials, which includes gypsum, metal, rubber, cotton and so on, is replaced or eliminated. The new generation of biological materials is built on the development basis of different fields, such as medical science, material science, physics. In the material science area, high polymer science that studies high molecular material is one of the most essential areas for medical applications. The representative material includes hydroxyapatite, collagen, polypeptide, polymethacrylate hydroxyethyl ester, fibrous protein, and so on. Compared with the previous generation, these materials have better mechanical and biochemical properties. In the physiological environment, these materials can replace and mimic the physiological functions of natural material in the human body after being implanted.

In the last two decades, with the application of gene technology, biological materials utilized many new theories in its development, such as growth factor, somatostatin, regulatory factor. So live cells begin to mingle with new biological materials to form bioactive material. The hybridization of living materials and artificial materials has been a promising direction in the 21st century.

According to different criteria, biomaterials can be divided into several groups. In different medical application, biomaterials include repair materials in several fields:

(1) In the bone-muscle system, biomaterials are used in bone, tooth, joint, tendon and so on;

(2) In the cardiovascular system, biomaterials are used in heart, cardiac valve, blood vessel and so on;

(3) In the medical disposal field, biomaterials are used in tissue adhesives, filtering membranes, suture lines and so on.

According to the biochemical reaction level, biomaterials include bioinert materials, bioactive materials, biodegradable materials and bioabsorbable materials. However, the most common classification method is assorting by using different types of materials, so biomaterials include metallic material, high molecular materials (polymers), ceramics, composite materials, and natural materials.

Friction and wear phenomena are very common in nature. Friction and wear always occur on the surfaces where two or more objects are in contact with each other and move relative to each other. Many parts of modern machinery consist of sliding and rolling surfaces that are greatly affected by friction and wear. About 1/3 to 1/2 of the energy produced by the industrial production sector in the world is consumed in various forms of friction and wear. The power, which is consumed by various types of friction and wear in a car, has reached about 30% of its effective power. For example, in the cylinder-liner-piston, the friction loss between the piston rings accounts for more than 40% of the total friction loss. According to the statistics of the United States in the year of 1997, the damage caused by mechanical equipment wear and friction occupied about 12% of the gross national product, which is equal to around 200 billion US dollars. If the knowledge of tribological theory is well used in the design to improve the friction and wear situation in various types of mechanical equipment in the engineering field, the economic cost and energy consumption would be effectively reduced in industrial production. Therefore, tribology has been put forward and become the focus of scientific research in various countries.

The definition of tribology was proposed by Dr. H. Peter Jost in 1966. He synthesized friction, wear and lubrication into an organic whole, forming a new discipline "tribology", and the English Department of Oxford has established a special English language for it, the term "Tribology". In 1973, world-renowned tribology scholars D. Dowson and V. Wright defined biotribology as a discipline that studies all tribological problems associated with biological systems (Dowson & Wright, 1973; Dowson, 1998). In 1967, the British Society of Mechanical Engineers and the Association of Prostheses jointly held the first international conference on lubrication and wear of natural and artificial joints, including the participation of many engineering experts, doctors and physicists. The meeting marked the beginning of the official study of biotribology. Biotribology research includes related research on organisms such as animals, plants and humans. The most in-depth and widely used research is the study of human biotribology. At present, most of the biotribology researches at home and abroad focus on human biotribology, which is of great significance for ensuring human health and improving the quality of life. Biotribology is an emerging edge discipline that combines the knowledge of medicine, physics, materials science, and engineering science to analyze and solve tribological problems.

Biotribology can be divided into human biotribology and animal bionic tribology. Human biotribology is the science of "researching all tribological problems associated with human biological systems". Human biotribology has its special research objects and theoretical systems in the human body. Its research objects include the following ones.

First, it studies the tribological mechanism of the friction pair formed between the living body and the living body in the human body, such as the joint surface between the joint surface of the joints, natural dentition and natural dentition, natural cornea and eyelids, organs and organs, muscles and muscles, muscles and bones, blood and blood vessel walls.

Second, the tribological problem of the friction pair formed between the human tissue and the artificial object is studied, that is, the tribological problem between the living body and the non-living body, for example, the tribological mechanism of natural and artificial dentures, eyelids and artificial corneas, blood and artificial blood vessels, stomach and esophageal wall and endoscopes, intestinal wall and food and feces, plantar skin and footwear, palm skin and tools. The purpose is to ensure that the surface of these artifacts does not harm human tissue, and to study the negative effects of human tissue and biological environment on the material of artificial objects.

Third, the tribological problem of artificial friction pairs in the human environment is studied. At this time, both sides of the friction pair are artificial materials. There are two types of artificial friction pairs directly or indirectly related to the human anatomical environment. The former is an artificial joint composed of metal and high molecular polyethylene, a bearing in an artificial heart, a prosthetic heart valve, *etc*. These friction pairs are directly working in the human body. Working in the environment, the latter is a friction pair working in the extracorporeal circulation system, such as bearings and valves that are in direct contact with blood in the extracorporeal blood circulation system. Although they are not located inside the human body, they are in contact with the internal tissues of the human body through the blood.

Fourth, it studies the friction pair formed between the surface of the natural and artificial organs and the medium. The medium includes liquid (such as joint synovial fluid), solid-liquid two-phase fluid (such as plasma and blood cells), and solid-liquid two-phase mixed slurry (such as chewing the food in the stomach). The research content includes the influence of interface friction on the flow of the medium; and the wear of the solid interface, especially the interface of the living body.

Comparing with the traditional tribology problems in the engineering field, many distinct properties can be found in the biotribology field. A pivotal problem always put forward in biotribology is biological activity or bioactivity. In artificial organs, artificial biomaterial will integrate with living organisms. If the bioactivity is not high enough, the bond between prosthesis and living organisms cannot be developed, and the surgery may fail in the future.

Another important factor that affects prosthesis is biocompatibility. Some biomaterials have better biological biocompatibility with the tissues and improve the tissue interface condition. In biotribology field, the self-adaptive ability and self-repair ability are also important. When some natural or artificial materials or organs have damages occurred, they have the capability to repair themselves on their own and can perform this process without any diagnosis of the damage or intervention of other people.

1.2   Biotribology of Organism Biomaterials

1.2.1   Biotribology *in Vitro*

In the course of biological evolution, organisms produce a variety of modes of movement and behavior. The most common biological movement for the animal body includes running, jumping, wriggling, tumbling, swimming and other ways. For plants, the plant itself undergoes slow movement during its growth and development, and plants need to absorb nutrients through the roots and ensure their attachment to the ground. The survival and development status of animals and plants on the earth has been formed by the survival of the fittest for a long time, which can be said to be the result of natural selection. The process leading to this result is directly related to the changes in the structural characteristics of animals and plants during their development and evolution. Changes in the structure of living organisms can lead to changes in the characteristics of living organisms and have a huge impact on their adaptation to the environment, which has always brought great enlightenment to the development of human science and technology. Outside the animal, it has evolved tissue, such as skin, hair, nails, feet, claws, scales, that can be in direct contact with the environment. These different organizations have different functions in life, but without exception, they are in mechanical contact with other surfaces in the environment. There are a lot of small scales on the surface of the snake, especially in the scales of the abdomen. The scales are arranged in a shingle shape. These scales act as abdominal scales to power the snakes under the contraction of the muscles. The contact relationship between snake scales and space determines that it has a good possibility in the walking process in a small space and is used in the field of robotics. Many terrestrial animals need the foot to provide support for the weight of the body during the movement, and also need to provide the driving force through the interaction between the foot and the ground. This driving force is alone in the early days. Take out and define it as friction. As a result, many terrestrial animals have relatively rough feet and strong feet on the feet for gripping various interfaces such as the ground, rocks and branches. For large mammals, due to the large size of the foot, its feet no longer play a huge role, the feet are close to the plane and have soft muscles to provide cushioning.

For animals that are good at climbing, such as goats and monkeys, their feet form a unique biotribological structure for climbing, which ensures sufficient grip and driving force. For invertebrates such as insects, their types and quantities are enormous. In the course of walking, camouflage, reproduction, and eating, insects form a unique body surface structure to cope with various dangers. They also follow the principles of biotribology. Without friction, they cannot survive in nature. The other two common types of frictional resistance are fish and bird activities. Fish swims with resistance to swimming and birds have air resistance during flight. These can also be linked to biotribology.

Another large number and variety of living things on earth are plants. Plants are generally fixed at a certain location and do not involve the friction of the foot during the movement. The root system of the plant needs to be bound and adhered to the soil to maintain the stability during the growth of the plant, and also needs to absorb a large amount of water and nutrients, so that there is also a frictional adhesion between the plant roots and the soil. Some researchers have studied the combination of plant roots and soil as a typical application of composite materials. The surface roughness of plant roots has a great effect on the binding ability of roots to the soil, which is conducive to maintaining the smoothness and compactness of the soil. In the study of the wax layer on the surface of plant leaves, for example, for ball orchids, green onions, and eggplants, it has been used as an environmentally friendly lubricant additive for industrial friction.

1.2.2   Biotribology *in Vivo*

Friction and wear inside the living body are also the study subject of biotribology. The study of friction in organisms include various joint friction problems, such as teeth, heart valves, blood vessels, esophagus, urethra, anus, bone tissue, surgical medical equipment.

In the study of friction in life, the longest research history and the most abundant research experience are artificial joints. At present, artificial joints have been widely used in clinical practice, and the lifespan of mainstream products has reached more than 20 years. Every year, there are 1–1.5 million patients in China that need a joint replacement. However, in actual use, the problem of artificial joint wear has been plaguing patients, and wear particles can cause various complications, which are all for artificial joints. Long-term use presents challenges.

Another key issue in life friction is the erosion of the heart valve and the resulting mechanical failure of the valve. There may be a screw pump or a vane pump in the artificial heart, and there are various friction pairs in the moving parts. Due to the current technical limitations of the artificial heart, the artificial heart is only used as a means of maintaining life before heart transplantation, cannot be used as a permanent transplant, and needs to continue to be improved in tribology design. For mammals, heart valves help blood flow into the heart in a fixed direction. The durability of the heart valve directly affects the life safety of the human body, and the failure probability can reach more than 3%. After the heart valve is implanted in the human body, the life of the cage is directly related to the life of the heart valve. The blood pressure difference in the heart acts directly on the heart valve and cage, so each year the heart valve and cage are subject to tens of millions of blood flow impacts. During this condition, the heart valve will be gradually destroyed and even cause valvular heart disease. At this point, the blood will flow in the wrong direction, or cause stenosis, which will threaten life.

The role of the teeth in the human body to cut and wear food is a typical biotribology tool. Dental defects often occur in the crowd, and as living standards increase, more and more people have dentures and dental implants, which will bring about the corresponding friction and wear problems. At the same time, the lubrication of saliva also plays a good role in the oral cavity, and the role of saliva in bio-friction needs further research.

Current contact lenses are already common, but the problem of friction between them and the eyeball has not been resolved. The human body glasses use the principle of fluid dynamic lubrication to achieve frictional contact. The surface friction coefficient can reach 0.005, but the contact lens increases the friction coefficient to more than 0.04, which is more than ten times that of the natural human eye, which will cause damage to the cornea. It also causes corneal hypoxia during the wearing of contact lenses.

1.3　Biotribology of the Human Body

Human beings and other animals have a variety of organs. Some organs in the human physiological process have to contact and slide each other, so these activities will produce different types of friction, and sometimes wear phenomena will take place. The design of the frictional parts of these organisms is natural, and it is selected by humans and animals in the long-term natural evolution. These organs always have excellent tribology properties. Some of these organs have better frictional properties and have far exceeded the performance of mechanical bearings designed by humans in many aspects. The human body is like a sophisticated mechanical system, where parts of the organs are the different parts that make up the system, and friction and wear behavior occur between different parts of the organs. The human body is supported by many bones, and the bones are connected by connective tissue and cartilage. These complicated connecting structures are called joints. The human joints contain different kinds of joints, including immobilized joints, less moving joints and moving joints, so these moving joints are also known as "synovial joints". The synovial joint is a kind of typical organ in the human physiological system. This kind of joint is used for human movement or supports the human body in many different areas, such as hip joints, knee and shoulder joints. The human joint system of the sliding joint in the human body is a typical organ that has many phenomena of friction, wear and tear. The basic structure of the sliding joint system is composed of three parts: joint surface, joint capsule and joint cavity. The joint surface is related to the cartilage. The relative movement occurs between the two joint surfaces. The joint capsule has the structure of connective tissue, but the joint capsule is a closed area. The secretion of the joint capsule is used as slip fluid which can keep the lubrication of the joint. The joint cavity also keeps the joint in a closed negative pressure state, and it keeps the joint movement stable and flexible. The fluid contains a lot of water, hyaluronic acid (HA) and mucus proteins, as well as a small number of lymphocytes and macrophages. The sliding joint system is abundant in both human and animal, and has good function in daily activities. The coefficient of friction of the human hip joint in motion reaches $0.01-0.03$, and the ankle of animals reaches $0.0044-0.0099$ (Wright & Dowson, 1976). In daily activities of people, the human body's moving joints, especially the lower limb joints, are subjected to strong axial pressure. The surface of the human joint is covered with several kinds of cartilage, this layer of cartilage tissue has a unique mechanical characteristic. This cartilage can disperse the pressure load of the joint surface and reduce the shock. Most importantly, they can reduce the friction coefficient of the joint surface. As a result, the joint system in the moving of the human body will have a very small wear for a long time living. Most joints of human beings can maintain safe operation and precise moving for 70 or 80 years without any significant damage on its surface (Hills, 1995). It is interesting that the characteristics of cartilage allow the joint to endure such a long duration and so powerful mechanical effects throughout life.

In the orthopedic clinic practices, various trauma caused by arthritis and car accidents can lead to joint system damage. As the disease progresses, it can cause joint deformity, pain and even loss of function, and it will cause various complications, causing huge losses to society and families. The American College of Rheumatology divides joint diseases into ten categories including more than 200 species, of which the first three are mostly arthritis. The first category is extensive connective tissue disease, such as rheumatoid arthritis; the second is arthritis associated with the spine, such as ankylosing spondylitis; the third category is osteoarthritis (OA). For joint diseases that are not treated by non-surgical treatment, artificial joint replacement is a safe, economical, and effective method to relieve pain and rebuild joint function. The so-called artificial joint replacement is to use artificial materials such as high-molecular polyethylene, cobalt-chromium-molybdenum alloy and ceramics with good biocompatibility, high mechanical strength and high wear resistance to make the joint head and joint surface instead of the original diseased joint. As a result, it can be easy to restore the joint to its original function.

Artificial joint replacement involves the comprehensive applications of multiple disciplines such as orthopedics, biomechanics, materials science, mechanics and computer science. Artificial joint replacement began in 1891 with the German Glunk using ivory to make the mandibular joint. The extensive development of artificial joint replacement was made in the early 1960s when Sir John Charnley proposed metal femoral head and high molecular polyethylene and combined hip joints. Charnley's joint prosthesis design is widely used due to its stability, low friction and low looseness. At present, there are many kinds of artificial joints, and the whole body of different joints can be replaced, such as artificial knee joint, artificial hip joint, artificial shoulder joint, artificial elbow joint and artificial knuckle joint. After decades of development in medical science, artificial joint materials have also evolved from the original natural materials to various metal materials, ceramic materials and polymer materials (Tengvall, Lundstrom, Freij-Larsson, Kober & Wesslen, 1993; Laing, Ferguson Jr. & Hodge, 1967; Friedrich, Karger-Kocsis, Sugioka & Yoshida, 1992; de Groot, 1993; Buly, Huo, Salvati, Brien & Bansal, 1992; Watters, Spedding, Grimshaw, Duffy & Spedding, 2005; Chiba, Sakakura, Kobayashi & Kusayanagi, 1997; Bothe, Beaton & Davenport, 1940; Liang, Shi, Fairchild & Cale, 2004; Suciu, Iwatsubo, Matsuda & Nishino, 2004). Metallic materials have good mechanical properties, in addition to joint surfaces and load-bearing components, including stainless steel, titanium alloys and cobalt-based alloys. Ceramic materials are divided into bioinert ceramics and bioactive ceramics. Alumina and zirconia are commonly used in joint components. Bioactive ceramics such as hydroxyapatite are used for metal surface treatment to enhance implant and natural bone bond strength. The polymer materials mainly include ultra-high molecular weight polyethylene

(UHMWPE) and polymethyl methacrylate (PMMA). The UHMWPE is used for the joint surface matched with the metal material, and the bone cement is used for fixing the joint parts and the natural bone of the human body.

According to the data of the Swiss Sulzer Plastic Surgery Company, there are 1.1 million hip joint implants every year in the world. There are 1.74 million potential cases in the Chinese mainland, and a large number of patients need artificial joint replacement every year because of accidents. About 30 million people worldwide have implanted various types of artificial joints, and in the United States alone, there are 500000 people undergoing artificial joint replacement surgery every year. In 1998, more than 50 international medical organizations and academic groups in Sweden proposed to set the year 2000 to 2010 as the "Decade of Bone and Joints". The main goal is to launch global medical experts to improve through basic and clinical research the quality of life of joint patients. China also has "Decade of Bone and Joints" from 2002 to 2012, that is, China's bones and health for 10 years.

In the human natural joint system, the joint surface has cartilage coverage, and the joint capsule secretes an appropriate amount of joint fluid as a lubricating fluid to form a good self-lubricating system. After the artificial joint is implanted, the original lubrication mechanism of the joint is destroyed. During human movement, the peak value of human joint stress ranges from 0.5 to 5 MPa (Brand, 2005), and the load reaches 4000 to 6000 N (Smith, 1972). Under the action of the human body load, with the prolongation of artificial joint use time, the artificial joint surface will wear and affect the realization of joint function. For example, artificial hip joint prosthesis mostly chooses UHMWPE as the bearing surface of the acetabulum. Because the polyethylene itself has low yield strength, the force is easy to deform, and a large number of abrasive grains will be generated in the long-term use of the joint. These abrasive grains will induce the body cells to produce a series of biological reactions that directly activate the osteoclasts to cause osteolysis around the prosthesis, causing aseptic loosening of the fixed prosthesis during surgery, which is one of the important factors that cause the failure of artificial joint replacement. Metal-to-metal artificial hip joints have problems such as stress shielding effect, the release of metal ions and metal particles. Metals form an oxide layer on the surface in an oxygen-rich environment in the human body. Metal ions and particles are released after the oxide layer is detached, and metal ions are potentially toxic to humans (Witzleb, Ziegler, Krummenauer, Neumeister & Guenther, 2006).

In order to solve the problems in the artificial joints and prolong the service time of the artificial joints, the researchers used various methods to improve joint materials (Bader, Steinhauser, Willmann & Gradinger, 2001; Han & Blanchet, 1997). Commonly used methods include improved joint design, modification of existing joint materials, the improved wear resistance of the pair, and development of new joint materials. Since 1970, Boutin *et al.* have applied alumina ceramics to hip arthroplasty, which has matured and been widely used over the decades (Sawae, Murakami & Chen, 1998; Fruh & Willmann, 1998). Ceramic materials have good wettability, which has a positive effect on the adsorption of the surface liquid film during exercise. Ceramic materials work well in wet environments, do not release metal ions, and have a minimum coefficient of friction (Banchet, Fridrici, Abry & Kapsa, 2007; Xiong & Ge, 2001). The ceramic material is hard and does not react chemically or corrode. However, the brittleness of ceramic materials is its Achilles heel. The fracture strength and tensile strength of ceramics are low, and the installation precise of the prosthesis is also required in use (Zichner & Willert, 1992; Agins, Alcock, Bansal, Salvati, Wilson Jr., Pellicci & Bullough, 1988).

The mechanical properties of hard artificial joint materials and natural joint materials are very different, which directly affects the life of artificial joints. Therefore, researchers have studied many new artificial joint materials, such as polyetheretherketone (PEEK), polyvinyl alcohol (PVA) hydrogel and polyvinylpyrrolidone (PVP) hydrogel (Bodugoz-Senturk, Macias, Kung & Muratoglu, 2009; Freeman, Furey, Love & Hampton, 2000; Lakouraj, Tajbakhsh & Mokhtary, 2005; Wu, Zhao, Wang & Zhang, 2008). Researchers began to consider artificial joint materials and designs from the perspective of natural joints, and Professor Dowson who is from the United Kingdom proposed a new concept of artificial joints—Cushion Joint (Dowson, 1990; Dowson & Wright, 1981; Dowson, 1989). Professor Dowson believes that natural joints have obvious liquid film characteristics. The key to improving the lubrication performance of artificial joints is to promote the realization of hydrodynamic lubrication in joints, which needs to be realized by a new material with low elastic modulus similar to natural articular cartilage. Therefore, while improving the traditional design, it is necessary to study the anti-wear mechanism of natural articular cartilage and to improve the wear resistance of artificial joints by simulating the structure and performance of natural articular cartilage. Studying the friction and wear properties of natural articular cartilage materials and exploring the mechanism of friction and wear of natural articular cartilage can not only further reveal the friction and wear mechanism of natural articular cartilage, but also have important significance for further improving the design of artificial joint materials and the life of artificial joints.

The friction causes of human tissue are essentially different from the friction mechanism in mechanical parts. The repeated friction of the lubricating film will cause physiological changes in the surface layer of the human body and frictional changes of the tissue, which are mechanical damage, physiological variation and self-repair of tissue. The combined results are related to human health and disease. The theoretical system of human biotribology includes a series of basic problems: friction surface and contact problems of human tissue, friction and lubrication mechanism of human tissue, wear and tear of human tissue, friction variation and self-repair, friction behavior and human environment, microscopic of human tissue dynamic interface and growth, friction flow and micro-exchange in the human body.

The human motor system consists of bones, joints and skeletal muscles, which together account for 60% of the total weight of the human body. There are more than 200 bones in adults. These different kinds of bones are usually connected by joints and ligaments to form a rigid bone scaffold to realize the physiological functions of the human body. Especially when bones are in the movement of the human body, they act as a lever, the joints are the movement hubs, and the skeletal muscles provide the power. The bone tissue is mainly composed of three parts: bone, bone marrow and periosteum. The bone includes the dense bone and the cancellous bone. The dense and compact bone has the ability to resist stress and constitute the outer layer of the bone. The cancellous bone is interwoven by a plurality of lamellae, which are arranged in a sponge shape. The pressure and tension direction are consistent and distributed with the interior of the bone. The periosteum is a membrane that is covered in the bone and construct outside of the bone, and is composed of fibrous connective tissue. The bone component includes organic components and inorganic components, the organic components include collagen fibers and an amorphous matrix, and the inorganic components are mainly hydroxyapatite crystals.

Bone-to-bone is connected by fibrous connective tissue. When the cartilage and bone can form a bone connection, the connection is called a joint or bone connection. According to different methods, it can be divided into direct connection and indirect connection. The indirect connection is also called joint or synovial joint, which is the most differentiated form of bone connection. According to the number of axes of motion, it is divided into uniaxial joints (such as flexion joints and axle joints), biaxial joints (such as elliptical joints, saddle joints and ball joints) and multiaxial joints (such as ankle joints and plane joints).

The synovial joint is an indirect connection in the bone connection. There is a synovial cavity between the opposite bone surfaces. There is synovial fluid, which generally has a large range of motion, and the opposite bone surfaces are connected by the surrounding connective tissue. Although the shape and movement of the synovial joints in different parts of the human body are different, the basic structure consists of three parts: the articular surface, the joint capsule and the joint cavity. The articular surface refers to two opposite bone surfaces in the joint, and the shapes between them are adapted to each other. The convex surface of the spherical shape is called the joint head, and the concave side is called the joint socket. The bone surface is covered with smooth and elastic cartilage, namely articular cartilage. The thickness of articular cartilage varies with age and location, with an average of 2-3 mm thick, which can withstand loads and reduce friction. There is synovial fluid between the articular surfaces to reduce the friction between the bone surfaces and to provide nutrients to the articular cartilage. A joint capsule is a membrane that encloses the joint cavity and wraps around the joint surface. The joint capsule can be divided into an outer surface fiber layer and an inner surface synovial layer. The fibrous layer contains parallel and intersecting connective tissue, which has a strong connection with the epicardium and is thickened at the junction with the tendon and ligament. The synovial layer is rich in blood vessels, loose and attached to the non-articular part. The synovial layer secretes a small amount of mucus called synovial fluid, which is a clear, colorless or yellow viscous liquid containing a small number of cells, which are mainly lymph, a large amount of water, HA and mucin. The fibrous layer and the synovial layer are closely attached and adhere to the edge of the articular cartilage. The joint cavity refers to the cavity enclosed by the synovial layer of the joint capsule and the articular cartilage. The synovial fluid in the cavity is under negative pressure, which is used to maintain the stability and flexibility of the joint.

The hip joint and the knee joint belong to the synovial joint. It is mainly composed of the distal femur, the proximal humerus and the tibia. The knee joint is the largest joint with the most complex structure and more chances of injury. There is ligament reinforcement around the joint capsule of the knee joint. The synovial membrane protrudes in the upper direction of the upper edge of the humerus, forming a supracondylar sac between the quadriceps tendon and the lower part of the femur. The articular surface of the medial and lateral femoral condyles is spherically convex, while the glenoid fossa of the humerus is shallow and not suitable for each other. In the joint, a meniscus composed of fibrocartilage is produced. When the joint is active, a smooth joint articular cartilage on the joint surface can maintain the good frictional performance of the joint under the lubrication of the joint fluid. At the same time, the articular cartilage can effectively absorb energy, relieve contact stress, and provide an effect similar to the elastic pad to protect the bone under the cartilage from being damaged. Excessive wear of cartilage itself, OA and trauma can lead to lesions of articular cartilage, causing joint pain and swelling, and joint deformities can occur, causing great pain to the patient. People who use the mirror can see the condition of cartilage wear.

1.4   Articular Cartilage System

Articular cartilage on the articular surface plays an important role in the synovial joint which is trying to achieve its physiological function. Articular cartilage directly carries the load in joint motion, providing good protection for the joint. Cartilage is a connective tissue composed of chondrocytes and interstitial cells. The cartilage matrix consists of fibrous components and non-fibrous components (amorphous matrix). Cartilage has more intercellular substance, or cartilage, than other common types of connective tissue. The matrix, which has a cavity (pit), in which there are chondrocytes, and the chondrocytes continuously synthesize the matrix to maintain the presence of the matrix. There are three types of cartilage: hyaline cartilage, elastic cartilage, and fibrocartilage. The fresh hyaline cartilage is blue-white and transparent, and the embryonic hyaline cartilage has a temporary scaffolding function, and then the scaffolding effect is replaced by bone. Adult hyaline cartilage is mainly distributed in the walls of the respiratory tract (trachea and bronchus), the sternal ends of the ribs, and the bone surface (articular cartilage) in the joints. Cartilage lacks blood vessels, nutrients are diffused from capillaries in nearby connective tissue, or provided by synovial fluid secreted by the joint capsule in the joint cavity. There are no lymphatic vessels and nerves in the cartilage, and the metabolic rate is low.

The matrix of articular cartilage is divided into formed and non-formed parts.

The tangible matrix is mostly collagen fiber and a small amount of elastin. The non-formation is mainly water and proteoglycan. Proteoglycans are obtained by combining amino dextran such as HA, chondroitin sulfate, keratan sulfate or the like with a specific protein. The long-chain core protein is combined with chondroitin sulfate and keratan sulfate as side chains, and then further forms a plurality of aggregates together with long-chain HA and glycoprotein containing sialic acid. This proteoglycan agglomerate has a large molecule and can bind to water, ensuring that the cartilage can resist the compressive stress load. Articular cartilage usually contains about 80% of total body weight, collagen fiber accounts for 60% of dry weight, and proteoglycans account for 30% of dry weight. Collagen fibers are structural macromolecules in the matrix, and their reticulated framework imparts tissue shape and tensile shear properties. The affinity of cartilage for water is mainly derived from proteoglycans. Since collagen is soft, the hardness of most cartilage tissues is formed by hydrophilic proteoglycans. Collagen fibers in cartilage are type II collagen fibers, which are characterized by the inability to form large bundle structures present in the tissue but are interlaced with proteoglycan macromolecules. The molecules of proteoglycans may bind to collagen fibers with weak chemical bonds. The collagen in the matrix is mainly in the form of fibrils, and its diameter is mostly sub-fibrous. The refractive index of the fiber is close to that of the surrounding amorphous interstitial (Trunfio-Sfarghiu, Berthier, Meurisse & Rieu, 2007).

1.5   Surface and Contact Observation of Articular Cartilage

Traditional scanning electron microscopy (SEM) is often used as an observation in early studies (Clark, 1991; Clark & Rudd, 1991; Akizuki, Mow & Muller, 1986; Bald & Robards, 1978; Bullough, Yawitz, Tafra & Boskey, 1985; Gardner, O'Connor & Oates, 1981; Clark, 1985; De Bont, Boering, Havinga & Liem, 1984; Dempsey & Bullivant, 1976; Ghadially, 1983). Since SEM is required for sample preparation, this will have an effect on the aqueous and non-conductive cartilage samples, which will change the appearance of the cartilage. The appearance of environmental scanning electron microscope (ESEM) compensates for the defects of SEM (Kjellsen & Jennings, 1996; Ali & Barrufet, 1995), which allows the cartilage to remain in its original state for observation, without the need to dry and spray the sample, which is even more conducive to the more accurate observation of cartilage surface. Graindorge, Ferrandez, Ingham, Jin, Twigg & Fisher (2006) have used SEM, ESEM and other methods to compare the knee joint wear and non-wear cartilage.

The cartilage surface is not smooth, has a certain roughness and affects the surface contact behavior in cartilage friction (Clarke, 1972). Many researchers have found that the cartilage surface is also rough in the test (Sayles, Thomas & Anderson, 1979; Chappuis, Sherman & Neumann, 1983), the surface roughness is often more than 10 microns, and the height distribution is close to the Gauss distribution. Under such roughness, the cartilage can be separated by the lubricating film during the mutual movement of the light load. But when the cartilage is under heavy load or impact load, the cartilage on both surfaces may be partially contacted, and the contact may be painful when the contact is severe.

For the measurement of the contact state of cartilage with other materials, there is currently no effective measurement method, only an indirect measurement is used. Hiroshi, Hasuo, Fuwa & Ikeuchi (2007) used frustrated total internal reflection (FTIR) to determine the light reflectance of the cartilage and lens contact surfaces. The researchers believe that due to the hydrophilicity of the proteoglycan, there is a layer of hydration on the surface of the cartilage and the mirror. The thickening of the layer reduces the friction, and the thickness of the layer is inversely proportional to the light reflectance. Therefore, the reflectance can be indirectly obtained from the measured reflectance. The thickness of the hydration layer changes, and finally the relationship between the friction coefficient and the contact state of the cartilage and the lens is established. It was found that the friction coefficient is directly proportional to the light reflectance. The closer the cartilage surface fiber is to the prism, the greater the reflectivity, so it is related to the friction coefficient due to the thickness of the hydrated liquid film. As shown in their papers, the film thickness of Region 1 is larger than the film thickness of Region 2, and more fibers in the cartilage surface layer in Region 2 reflect the light, and as a result, the reflectance of Region 2 is larger than that of Region 1. Kobayashi & Oka (2001, 2003) and Kobayashi, Toguchida & Oka (2001) have used laser confocal microscopy to observe the contact state of rabbit articular cartilage with the glass surface. During the test, the physiological load of the rabbit was applied and lubricated with physiological saline, and the contact zone was divided into the contact zone and the liquid pool zone, and it was considered that the liquid film was loaded between the two zones.

1.6　Biomechanical Properties of Articular Cartilage

The thickness of the articular cartilage varies with age and joint position. It is not easy to cut the cartilage specimen. The indentation test is often used for the study of the mechanical properties of articular cartilage. The indentation test is the most widely accepted and the most widely used (Hoch, Grodzinsky & Koob, 1983; Hori & Mockros, 1976; Athanasiou, Agarwal, Muffoletto, Dzida, Constantinides & Clem, 1995; Elmore, Sokoloff, Norris & Carmeci, 1963; Athanasiou, Rosenwasser, Buckwalter, Malinin & Mow, 1991; Froimson, Ratcliffe, Gardner & Mow, 1997; Altman, Tenenbaum & Latta, 1984; Coletti Jr., Akeson & Woo, 1972; Sokoloff, 1961; Mow & Lai, 1979). Bar and Gocke first studied the relationship between indentation depth and time using the indentation test method. Sokoloff (1963) has suddenly pressed into the cartilage layer with constant weight and recorded the relationship between the depth of the indenter pressed into the cartilage and the time. Under the condition that the cartilage was a linear isotropic incompressible body, the elastic modulus of the material is obtained by the elastic mechanic solution.

$$E = \frac{P}{2.67W_0a},$$

where P is the applied load, W_0 is the initial indentation depth, and a is the indentation radius.

Considering that the cartilage is only a thin layer, Hayes, Keer, Herrmann & Mockros (1972) corrected the calculation formula, and they derived the formula as follows:

$$E = \frac{P(1 - v^2)}{2W_0ak(a/h, v)},$$

where v is the Poisson's ratio, $k(a/h, v)$ is the correction factor, which is a function of the ratio of the radius of the indentation to the thickness h of the cartilage layer and the Poisson's ratio. This correction factor has been used for the examination. Cartilage has multiple layers and biphasic properties, which makes it difficult for researchers to establish accurate cartilage indentation test models. Researchers often use linear elastic basic rules to describe test results, and later gradually establish complex mathematical models (Lu, Sun, Guo, Chen, Lai & Mow, 2004; Mak, Lai & Mow, 1987; Mow, Gibbs, Lai, Zhu & Athanasiou, 1989).

Non-limiting compression tests and restrictive compression tests are also commonly used to study the biomechanical properties of cartilage. In the non-restrictive compression test, the cartilage specimen was compressed by two impervious plates, and Young's modulus of the cartilage compression direction was obtained according to the stress-strain curve (Jurvelin, Buschmann & Hunziker, 1997; Wong, Ponticiello, Kovanen & Jurvelin, 2000; Wang, Deng, Ateshian & Hung, 2002). In the restrictive compression test, the cartilage was placed in a rigid chamber that was impervious to water and compressed with a rigid permeable plate, and the upper portion of the sample was freely drained. Since the sample is radially deformed, the water in the cartilage can only flow through the axial direction, thereby determining the two-phase properties of the cartilage (Schinagl, Gurskis, Chen & Sah, 1997; Armstrong & Mow, 1982). For example, Setton, Zhu & Mow (1993) performed a restrictive compression test on the cartilage pin, and the cartilage pin was pre-treated, which was divided into two parts: the removal of the surface layer and the absence of removal. The results showed that the friction and compression properties of the cartilage were changed after the cartilage surface was removed. As a result, the low permeability of the cartilage surface limits the loss of liquid in the matrix and increases the load carrying capacity of the liquid.

In daily life, articular cartilage in the human body is subjected to contact stress of 0-20 MPa at a frequency of 0.1-10 Hz. When people are running after the previous walking, the surface of the joints swiftly passes over certain areas of its surface, and the pressure of the contact area between the joint surfaces can quickly reach a large value from zero and then return to zero again. At this time, a very high hydrostatic pressure is generated in the interstitial fluid of the cartilage, and the conduction of pressure is achieved. MRI has been used to assess changes in cartilage volume and thickness produced by different physiological movements due to fluid exudation and tissue pyknosis leading to thinning of the entire cartilage (Eckstein, Reiser, Englmeier & Putz, 2001; Waterton, Solloway, Foster, Keen, Gandy, Middleton, Maciewicz, Watt, Dieppe & Taylor, 2000). The results of Eckstein, Lemberger, Stammberger, Englmeier & Reiser (2000) showed that the thickness of the cartilage layer of the tibiofemoral surface was reduced by about 2.8% after 30 times of knee flexion, and the thickness of the cartilage layer was 4.9% after going through the squat exercise of about 90 degrees squat movement.

The mechanical model of articular cartilage has also undergone a long development. Initial articular cartilage was considered a single-phase material (Hayes, Keer, Herrmann & Mockros, 1972; Sokoloff, 1966; Kempson, Spivey, Swanson & Freeman, 1971; Parsons & Black, 1977), and researchers often used indentation tests to measure (Sokoloff, 1966; Kempson, Freeman & Swanson, 1971). This model describes the mechanical properties of articular cartilage in static and equilibrium conditions, but does not describe the creep and stress relaxation of articular cartilage. Later, a viscoelastic model consisting of springs and bumpers was used to describe articular cartilage (Parsons & Black, 1977; Hayes & Mockros, 1971; Hayes & Bodine, 1978; Spirt, Mak & Wassell, 1989; Parsons & Black, 1979; Woo, Simon, Kuei & Akeson, 1980). For example, Hori & Mockros (1976) studied cartilage as a viscoelastic material and obtained the shear modulus of the rabbit femur at the indentation. Although such models can describe the creep and stress relaxation properties of cartilage, they cannot describe the flow of fluid in articular cartilage. The flow of fluid in the gap is closely related to the biomechanical properties of the tissue. The creep and stress relaxation behavior are due to the fluid flowing out of the cartilage surface and redistributing inside the tissue.

With the development of continuum theory, Mow, Kuei, Lai & Armstrong (1980) first used the theory of continuous medium mixing for the study of biological tissues, especially the study of cartilage, called two-phase theory, which regarded cartilage as being incompressible and immiscible. For the porous solid phase and liquid phase composition, the constitutive relationship is obtained as follows:

$$t^{(s)} = -\phi^{(s)} pI + \lambda_s tr(\varepsilon)I + 2\mu_s \varepsilon,$$

$$t^{(f)} = -\phi^{(f)} pI - \frac{2}{3}\mu_f \mathrm{div} v^f I + 2\mu_f D$$

momentum equation

$$-p^{(f)} = p^{(s)} = p\nabla\phi^{(f)} + K(v^{(f)} - v^{(s)}),$$

where s and f represent the solid phase and the liquid phase, respectively, $\phi^{(\alpha)}$ is the constitutive ratio, μ_s and λ_s represent the classical Lame elastic constant of the solid, μ_f is the liquid phase viscosity and ε is linear deformation of the solid. The porous solid phase has elasticity, the liquid phase penetrates in the solid phase, and frictional resistance occurs during the infiltration process, which is related to the viscoelasticity of the structure. In response to the observed effects of various ions in articular cartilage, Mow, Lai & Holmes (1982) and Lai, Hou & Mow (1991) proposed a three-phase theory, which developed a two-phase theory to explain the ion-induced expansion and the two-phase deformation.

The most widely used two-phase numerical analysis of articular cartilage is the finite element method. Spilker, Suh, Vermilyea & Maxian (1990) proposed a formula for the calculation of cartilage finite element. Soltz & Ateshian (2000) used two-phase mixing theory and CLE (Concise Linear Elasticity) theory to study the mechanical properties of cartilage to obtain the pressure between cartilage gaps. Wilson, Donkelaar, Rietbergen & Huiskes (2005) proposed a finite element model of porous viscoelastic fiber reinforcement and calculated the stress and strain of the fiber. In recent years, with the improvement of commercial finite element software, some researchers have applied commercial finite element software for research. The most widely used method is to study the mechanical behavior of cartilage using the content of consolidation theory. Graindorge, Ferrandez, Jin, Ingham & Fisher (2006) applied the ABAQUS software to study the liquid phase bearing and flow of the cartilage surface layer using consolidation theory. Pawaskar, Jin & Fisher (2007) used ABAQUS software to study the sliding of different states of cartilage and explained the calculation results by two-phase theory.

1.7 Lubrication Performance of Joints

The synovial joints of humans and animals have good frictional properties, and most of them can work normally for more than 70 years, which is mainly manifested by low friction and low wear between articular cartilage on the articular surface. Many researchers have performed friction tests on the joints of humans and certain animals through various forms of devices.

To explore the lubrication mechanism of natural joints, researchers have put forward many hypotheses. The most famous ones are the fluid dynamic lubrication theory proposed by MacConaill *et al.*, the boundary lubrication theory proposed by Charnley *et al.*, the elastic fluid dynamic lubrication theory proposed by Dowson *et al.*, the extrusion film lubrication theory proposed by Fein *et al.*, and the lifting lubrication theory proposed by Maroudas *et al.*

(1) Wedge Film Fluid Lubrication

The lubrication state of the joints was originally mentioned in Reynolds fluid lubrication theory. Dumbleton (1981) was influenced by Reynolds lubrication theory, combined with the study of sliding bearings in engineering, proposed in 1932 that the main lubrication mechanism of human natural joints is hydrodynamically lubricated and that the difference in diameter between the two joint surfaces is sufficient to form a bearing. The wedge-shaped space of the surface of the bearings can keep the film thickness. However, the formation of a wedge fluid lubrication requires a considerable sliding speed, which is inconsistent with the motion state of the joint. Dowson & Wright (1981) derived the formula for hydrodynamic lubrication when the ball is in contact with the plane, and the calculated result is too small compared to the roughness of the joint.

(2) Boundary Lubrication Theory

The relative movement speed between the articular surfaces is small, the active load is large, and the movement mode is a reciprocating motion mode. Charnley (1960) measured the coefficient of friction of the joint by using the ankle joint and found that the coefficient of friction of the joint does not change with speed. Therefore, he believed that the frictional resistance is independent of the speed. He found that the lubrication state between the joint surfaces should be the boundary lubrication. When the human joint is stationary for a period of time under load, any form of fluid lubrication film may not be present. At present, many scholars believe that boundary lubrication is the main lubrication method of joints. For example, Hills (2000) introduced the boundary lubrication problem of joints.

(3) Elastic Hydrodynamic Lubrication

The cartilage elastic modulus of the joint surface is very low, and it will undergo large deformation under the influence of the load during the movement. So, it may be elastic fluid dynamic lubrication. Unsworth (1995) first calculated the minimum film thickness of the joint surface using the theory of elastic flow and obtained a minimum lubricating film thickness of 0.1 μm on the joint surface. In 1978, Hamrock derived the ball close to the plane, and the minimum elastic film thickness of the low elastic modulus material was 1.02 μm, which is close to the surface roughness of the articular cartilage, indicating that the human joint may be in elastic hydrodynamic lubrication when the load is small.

(4) Squeeze Membrane Fluid Lubrication

The change of the film thickness of the joint during the movement requires a certain time. The film thickness established by the joint at high speed and light load will contribute to the lubrication under low speed and heavy load conditions, which is the concept of squeeze film lubrication. Fein derived the formula for calculating the joint extrusion film thickness, which Unsworth, Dowson & Wright (1975) verified the results by experiments.

(5) Exudation Lubrication and Lifting Lubrication

Exudation lubrication was proposed by McCutchen (1962). The main point is that articular cartilage acts as a porous substance, filled with liquid, as the cartilage deforms under load. The liquid in the cartilage space will penetrate into the joint surface, thus improving the joint. So, the friction surface may produce fluid lubrication. In contrast to exudation lubrication, the lifting lubrication proposed believed that when the articular cartilage is squeezed against each other, small molecules such as water in the synovial fluid in the cartilage enter the cartilage through the pores of the cartilage, and macromolecules such as HA are in the synovial fluid (Unsworth, 1995). The composition is trapped on the cartilage surface, increasing the viscosity of the synovial fluid, thereby increasing the fluid film thickness of the joint on the friction surface; in extreme cases, the synovial fluid can be squeezed into a gelatinous substance, thereby improving the load carrying capacity of the boundary membrane. When the two articular cartilage surfaces are in contact, a small space is formed between the two surfaces which are relatively closed with synovial fluid. The pressure on the surface will be greater than the pressure in the cartilage. The pressure will spread from the cartilage surface to the inside, so the small molecular weight substance will get through the cartilage surface into the cartilage matrix.

The above various joint lubrication hypotheses cannot explain the lubrication state of the joint separately. The contact area between the cartilage on the joint surface is irregular, and the load and movement state of the joint are also constantly changing. Therefore, during the joint movement, there are usually several kinds of lubrication. The state works at the same time. Unsworth, Dowson & Wright (1975) found that in experimental research when the joint is subjected to sudden loading, the joint surface is in the state of squeeze film lubrication; when the joint is lightly loaded, the joint surface is in hydrodynamic lubrication state; when the load is applied, the joint surface is in a boundary lubrication state.

1.8   Repair of Articular Cartilage

To reconstruct the joint function, the damaged cartilage must be repaired. The current methods mainly include two methods of tissue engineering cartilage and artificial joint material.

1.8.1 Tissue Engineering Cartilage

Tissue engineering is the comprehensive use of the basic principles of biology, engineering, and medicine to create biological alternatives or to promote the repair of lost or defective tissues. In specific operations, different pathways are used to utilize cells, biomaterial scaffolds, and regulatory factors. The bioreactor or implanted functional tissue generated *in vivo* is used *in vitro*. Tissue engineering combines the latest technologies in materials science, cell biology, molecular biology, medicine, and engineering technology, and uses engineering science and life science principles to develop biological substitutes that repair, maintain or improve tissue function. It will be ultimately achieving artificial joints. The purpose of tissue engineering materials is to replace, repair or enhance the function of tissues or organs (Mow & Huiskes, 2004). OA and joint degenerative diseases are common orthopedic diseases. They are mostly caused by joint wear, trauma or joint degeneration. The range of joint degeneration includes localized defects or large areas of cartilage surface erosion. The emergence of these diseases has triggered a demand for tissue-engineered cartilage. In 1968, Chestreman *et al.* injected a chondrocyte suspension into the defect of the articular cartilage. The defect was found to be synovial fibroblast repair, and a small number of neonatal chondrocyte nodules were found. In 1977, Green *et al.* proposed to find a suitable scaffold material. Inoculation of cartilage on it may form a good tissue repair, use a decalcified bone as a scaffold, inoculate the isolated chondrocytes and transplant them to the defect site (Green Jr., 1977). Cartilage tissue engineering research has developed rapidly in recent years and has become one of the hotspots in the field of international organization engineering research. The current research is mainly in the animal testing stage, and foreign countries have initially applied the results in clinical practice. The current main research contents include research on seed cells, selection of suitable seed cells; separation, culture and amplification of cells; manufacture and use of extracellular matrix; cell implantation techniques and use of growth factors; preclinical and clinical efficacy methods of observation and evaluation.

With the aging of the population and the improvement of living standards, there is a great demand for tissue engineering cartilage in the clinic. At present, tissue engineering is still in the early stage of development. Many problems need to be solved in order to achieve the clinical effective application. For example, the scaffold materials used in tissue engineering lack bearing capacity, and the connection mode and connection strength of tissue engineering cartilage and bone tissue need to be further improved. The long-term growth pattern of cartilage is also uncontrollable (Mahmood, Shastri, Blitterswijk, Langer & Riesle, 2005). In short, there is still a lot of work to be done before tissue engineering can solve cartilage diseases.

1.8.2   Artificial Joint Material

Artificial joint materials are mainly divided into metal materials, polymer materials, ceramic materials and composite materials. Metal materials mainly include stainless steel, cobalt-based alloys, titanium and titanium alloys, as well as memory alloys and other precious metals. Stainless steel materials were first used in the manufacture of artificial joints. Wiles first used stainless steel to make the femoral head and acetabulum during joint replacement surgery. Stainless steel materials have problems such as crevice corrosion, friction corrosion and fatigue corrosion in the physiological environment, so they are gradually replaced by cobalt-based alloys and titanium alloys, which are widely used in the manufacture of artificial joints. The use of polymer materials began in the 1940s. Polymer materials are widely used for their excellent physical and chemical properties. Commonly used polymer materials include UHMWPE, silicone rubber, polymethyl methyl acrylate (PMMA), PTFE, and PEEK. Silicone rubber is commonly used in artificial knuckles, and UHMWPE is widely used in artificial hip joints and artificial knee joints. Ceramic artificial joint materials mainly include alumina, zirconia, hydroxyapatite bioactive ceramics and bioactive glass. Ceramic materials have high strength, good wear resistance, strong chemical stability and corrosion resistance. Ceramic materials have some disadvantages, such as high hardness, high brittleness and high modulus of elasticity. A composite material is a novel material composed of two or more different materials, including polymer matrix composite, metal matrix composite, and ceramic composite. Biocomposites open up a broader field for the development of artificial joints, and biocomposites are still in the early laboratory research stage.

Traditional artificial joint materials are metal and non-metal materials with high elastic modulus. The mechanical properties, especially the elasticity of these materials, are far from the natural joints, which directly affect the life of artificial joints. Joint designs currently used in the field of artificial joints are difficult to achieve a life expectancy of more than 20 years. After decades of development, traditional hard joint materials were not effectively improved in the last century. In recent years, many new hydrogel-like artificial cartilage materials have emerged, including alginate gel, fibrin gel, HA gel, collagen gel, alginate gel, PVA hydrogel gels and chitosan gels (Kobayashi, Toguchida & Oka, 2003; Radice, Brun, Cortivo, Scapinelli, Battaliard & Abatangelo, 2000; Eyrich, Brandl, Appel, Wiese, Maier, Wenzel, Staudenmaier, Goepferich & Blunk, 2007). PVA hydrogel is recommended as an artificial cartilage material, which is prepared by processing a water-soluble polymer PVA by a certain method. PVA hydrogel has excellent biocompatibility, high elasticity and flexibility. Its macromolecules are cross-linked to form a porous network structure, which has a two-phase property similar to that of natural cartilage. It is regarded as an excellent artificial cartilage material in the field (Freeman, Furey, Love & Hampton, 2000; Pan, Xiong & Ma, 2007).

1.9　Friction in Joint Replacement

Artificial joints are joint prostheses made of medical biomaterials with good biocompatibility, high mechanical strength and high wear resistance. At present, the commonly used materials are mainly high molecular polyethylene, cobalt-chromium molybdenum alloy, ceramics and so on. Artificial joint prostheses that are made of artificial materials are used to replace diseased joints, to achieve joint function reconstruction, to relieve joint pain, to correct joint deformities, to maintain joint stability and to repair limb length. In particular, artificial joints can improve the quality of life for patients with joint disease in various situations. With the continuous development of materials science and medical technology, the field of artificial joint replacement has been expanded, which includes hip joints, knee joints, elbow joints, shoulder joints, wrist joints, metacarpophalangcal joints, interphalangeal joints and ankle joints. But the most mature and most widely used artificial joint field are artificial hip joints and artificial knee joints, accounting for about 90% of all cases of artificial joint replacement.

1.9.1　Artificial Hip Joint

Current hip arthroplasty is divided into hemiarthroplasty and total hip arthroplasty. Among them, hemiarthroplasty has developed earlier, and total hip arthroplasty has been widely used in the past ten years. Total hip replacement (THR) technology is more common. The total hip prosthesis consists of a metal handle, a femoral ball head, a cup and a cup liner. The metal handle is inserted into the upper half of the femoral medullary cavity and remains fixedly coupled. The ball head replaces the head of the femoral head and can be made of metal or ceramic. The cup and cup liner replace the hip socket. The cup material is metal and the inner liner can be made of polyethylene, ceramic or metal.

The semi-hip replacement can be divided into a monopolar artificial femoral head replacement, a bipolar artificial femoral head replacement, and a femoral head surface replacement. Unipolar artificial femoral head replacement is the use of bone cement to fix the prosthesis to a femoral head that has been trimmed to a hemisphere. In order to reduce the occurrence of prosthesis loosening and various dislocation, the inner surface of the cup is often designed to be cylindrical, or a short stem inserted into the femoral neck is added behind the cup. Bipolar artificial femoral head replacement is the addition of a metal acetabular cup and polyethylene pad in the outer layer of the artificial femoral head. The hip joint activity is loaded between the artificial femoral head/polyethylene pad and the acetabular metal cup and acetabulum.

Compared with a THR, the semi-hip has shorter operation time, less surgical trauma, better stability of the hip joint, and less postoperative complications. For young patients with femoral head necrosis, due to a large amount of activity, there is currently no surgery that can solve the problem for life. Doctors advocate a transitional treatment with low trauma and low cost before THR. Unipolar artificial femoral head replacement and bipolar artificial femoral head replacement for hemiarthroplasty are often used. After the half-hip replacement, due to the wear of the semi-replacement material and cartilage, the acetabular cartilage undergoes progressive degeneration, resulting in hip pain. Patients often need to undergo surgery for revision to THR.

1.9.2   Artificial Knee Replacement

In 1951, Walldius designed the first generation of hinged artificial knee joints, which achieved 110 degrees of improved joint flexion and extension, and uniaxial motion. The prosthetic material was acrylate. By the 1960s, the use of bone-fixed fully-restricted knee joints began to be applied, and the material was developed from the original stainless steel to a cobalt-based alloy. In the 1970s, semi-restricted artificial knee joints began to be applied. This type of joint provides a greater range of motion for the artificial knee joint based on the stability of the original restraint. The typical representative is the semi-restricted total knee prosthesis designed by Matthews and Kamfer of the United States. In 1973, John N. Insall introduced the cement-fixed total condylar knee, which brought the artificial knee into a new phase. The full knee has become the gold standard for evaluating dozens of artificial knee prostheses. The 15-year follow-up has a prosthesis retention rate of 94%. It is therefore known by many as the father of modern artificial knee joints. Gunston of the United Kingdom invented a multi-center artificial knee prosthesis with stainless steel or cobalt alloy and high molecular polyethylene as the articular surface, and cemented prosthesis with bone cement, and achieved good results. The metal/ultra-high molecular weight polyethylene joint combination has since been further developed into Freeman's "in-slot rolling" design. The artificial total knee prosthesis consists of three parts. The first part is a femoral prosthesis, which is made of a smooth alloy and can be combined with the lower end of the femur after special osteotomy to form the femoral articular surface. The second part is the tibial plateau prosthesis. There are two parts, the upper part is a layer of UHMWPE joint surface, the bottom is a metal disk with a handle to drag it, and the handle of the metal disk is inserted into the medullary cavity and tightly combined with the tibia. The third part is the tibial prosthesis, which is also composed of UHMWPE, which replaces the tibial articular surface and the tibia for tight integration.

After the artificial joint prosthesis is implanted into the human body, the complex motion form of the knee joint itself is required to bear the human body load, and the mounting surface and the mating surface of the joint prosthesis are worn due to friction. With daily use, the relatively soft UHMWPE material shows progressive wear and wear debris, which enters the gap around the prosthesis and is stimulated by local cells to stimulate the release of intercellular mediators. Production of tissue cell metabolic byproducts, which in turn recruits and activates local osteoclasts, promotes bone resorption around the prosthesis, causes bone loss, and ultimately causes aseptic loosening of the prosthesis (Blunn, Joshi, Minns, Lidgren, Lilley, Ryd, Engelbrecht & Walker, 1997; Insall, Scott & Ranawat, 1979).

The initial knee arthroplasty did not include patella replacement. The humeral replacement was first introduced in the 1970s. It reduced postoperative anterior knee pain, but also caused osteonecrosis, joint instability, ligament rupture and humerus. With the advancement of surgical techniques and the improvement of prosthesis design, the clinical effect of patella replacement has been significantly improved, but the debate about whether or not to perform patella replacement continues to this day. For the patient, the tibia is more physiological and anatomical than the humeral prosthesis. Complications increased significantly after patella replacement and a series of new complications occurred. Researchers who advocate patella replacement believe that although the patient's own tibia is more physiologically and anatomically normal on the joint, after knee replacement, the articular surface and mechanical properties change, and the movement of the tibia also changes, which affects the effect after replacement. Moreover, long-term contact and relative frictional movements of the tibial cartilage and metal joints can lead to various adverse effects (Komistek, Dennis, Mabe & Walker, 2000; Stiehl, Komistek, Dennis & Keblish, 2001), which can cause damage to the tibial cartilage and worsen over time (Burnett & Bourne, 2003; Shih, Shih, Wong & Hsu, 2004).

Chapter 2

Composition and Structure of Articular Cartilage and Preparation and Observation of Samples

2.1 Introduction

Artificial joints, which are designed to restore lost joints, have been widely used clinically. At present, artificial joints can be used for more than 20 years. It can eliminate joint pain and restore joint mobility. After surgery, patients can walk, climb stairs and exercise like normal people. At the same time, many young patients have begun artificial joint replacement, which puts higher requirements on the wear resistance of joints. At the same time, after joint replacement, there are many postoperative complications that are directly related to joint wear, such as osteolysis caused by high-molecular polyethylene wear particles, which in turn causes loosening of the prosthesis and acetabular wear. Natural joints maintain their excellent friction properties and are directly related to the composition of articular cartilage (Wright & Dowson, 1976; Tengvall, Lundstrom, Freij-Larsson, Kober & Wesslen, 1993). In order to improve the wear resistance of artificial joints, the structural characteristics and anti-wear properties of articular cartilage should be analyzed, and then the advantages and characteristics of the joints should be absorbed to develop artificial joints with better performance.

2.2 Preparation of Natural Cartilage Samples

In this subject, natural articular cartilage samples were obtained from human and animal knee joints, and the selected animal knee joint was the knee joint of adult healthy cattle. The bovine cartilage sample was obtained from the fresh femur knee joint femur. The cow was 18 months old, the joint was obtained within 12 hours after slaughter, and the cartilage sample was obtained within one hour after the joint was opened. There are two types of cartilage samples, one is a cartilage pin sample and the other is a cartilage piece sample. The cartilage pin sample is sampled by a hollow drill; the pin sample has a diameter of 9 to 11 mm, and the lower part of the sample retains about 4 mm of the matrix bone. The cartilage piece sample was obtained by cutting the joint surface by hand saw, and the flat surface was taken when cutting so that the bottom surface of the cartilage block was parallel and the surface, a cartilage block sample of about 30 mm in length and 20 mm in width, was obtained. During the processing of the cartilage sample, the cartilage surface is always washed with physiological saline to maintain the natural wet state of the cartilage. The sample is taken out, immersed in physiological saline, quickly placed in a refrigerator at −20 °C for freezing, and thawed two hours before the test. The human cartilage samples were obtained from human cadaveric knee femur surface cartilage. The corpses were male, aged 20–30 years old. The processing method of human cartilage samples was the same as that of bovine cartilage samples.

2.3   Preparation of Artificial Cartilage Samples

2.3.1   Common Methods for Preparing PVA Hydrogel

To improve joint life and reduce friction, damaged cartilage can be replaced by a low modulus of elasticity material similar to natural articular cartilage. Among the new artificial cartilage materials, PVA hydrogel is a porous elastic polymer material with good biocompatibility and no toxic side effects on the human body. It is considered to be an ideal artificial cartilage material.

PVA hydrogel has a variety of processing methods, and different methods have an effect on the properties of the hydrogel after processing. The PVA hydrogel previously made by conventional methods have low strength and have been improved in various ways.

(1) Physical Cross-Linking Method

PVA hydrogel has been proposed for biomedical applications by physical cross-linking as early as 1973. This method has been described in U.S. Patent No. 3875302 (Inoue, 1975), issued to 1975, to the preparation of PVA hydrogel by freezing the PVA aqueous solution at −5 °C. At present, the methods commonly used are "repeated freezing method" and "freezing-partial dehydration method". The repeated freezing method is to first configure the PVA aqueous solution, and then freeze it at $-10\ ^\circ\text{C}--40\ ^\circ\text{C}$ for a period of time, preferably at room temperature to form a physically crosslinked PVA hydrogel. The PVA hydrogel obtained by the repeated freezing method at normal temperature can maintain a gel state and has good elasticity and mechanical strength. In order to further improve the performance of the PVA hydrogel and increase the number of repeated freezing, a certain effect can be achieved. The freeze-partial dehydration method is to freeze the prepared PVA aqueous solution, put it into a vacuum for dehydration operation, and dehydrate it by 10%–20%. The obtained hydrogel was again immersed in water, the water content of the hydrogel was restored, and the basic properties remained unchanged.

The exact mechanism of physical cross-linking is controversial, and three models have been proposed to explain the mechanisms, which include direct hydrogen bonding, direct crystallite formation, and liquid-liquid phase separation followed by gelation. The first two models consider gel formation to separate through the nucleus and the growth phase, and the third assumes the process of phase separation as a metastable decomposition. Hydrogen bonding forms nodes and crystallites to form large polymer crystals. When the PVA aqueous solution is rapidly cooled, its viscosity increases. The molecular chain activity rapidly decreases and freezes, and the macromolecular chain does not respond to external conditions to form a crystalline structure; when thawed at room temperature, a small number of cells can move at room temperature. It can be readjusted to make the crystal structure obtained after refreezing more perfect, which further promotes the rearrangement of molecules in the system. It can strengthen the intermolecular interaction force (such as hydrogen bonding), and promote the improvement of the mechanical properties of the hydrogel . Okazaki, Hamada, Fujii, Mizobe & Matsuzawa (1995) considered that the PVA solution formed a microcrystalline structure during the freezing and thawing process, and the microcrystalline structure formed a cross-linking point to obtain a three-dimensional porous gel.

(2) Chemical Cross-Linking Method

This method uses a chemical cross-linking agent to chemically cross-link molecular chains under certain conditions to form a hydrogel. There are two ways of cross-linking, that is, forming a three-dimensional network by covalent bonds or coordination bonds. The chemical cross-linking agents used in the covalent bond mode mainly include glutaraldehyde, boric acid, epichlorohydrin, *etc.* (Hirai,

Maruyama, Suzuki & Hayashi, 1992; Bo, 1992). There are two ways to do this. One is to chemically cross-link a certain concentration of aqueous PVA solution with a chemical cross-linking agent, and the other is to directly immerse the gel obtained by physical cross-linking into a chemical cross-linking agent solution. The method used by the coordination bond method is that a PVA aqueous solution is complexed with a divalent metal salt to form a gel. Hyon, Cha & Ikada (1989) and Cha, Hyon, Oka & Ikada (1996) proposed an improved method of chemical cross-linking, and Trieu & Qutubuddin (1995) developed a method to obtain an improved chemical cross-linking method. The method dissolves PVA in a mixed solvent of dimethyl sulfoxide (DMSO) and water at a certain temperature, cross-links PVA with DMSO, and replaces DMSO in the sample with water or alcohol after cross-linking. Thereby, it can be avoiding the effect of DMSO on the human body, and the PVA hydrogel obtained by this method has better mechanical properties.

(3) Radiation Cross-Linking Method

The radiation cross-linking method is a PVA hydrogel obtained by irradiating an aqueous PVA solution with various rays, ultraviolet rays, electron beams or X-rays, or by physical cross-linking. During the irradiation of the PVA aqueous solution, the polymer molecules in the solution are cross-linked by free radicals, and the radiation cross-linking and radiation cracking occur simultaneously in the solution, wherein the radiation cross-linking is dominant. So, the cross-linking degree is proportional to the radiation dose. As the radiation increases, the concentration of PVA aqueous solution has a great influence on the cross-linking and degradation in gel production (Wang, Mukataka, Kokufuta & Kodama, 2000). By adjusting the amount of radiation dose, the water content, cross-link density and pore size of the PVA hydrogel will change accordingly. The PVA hydrogel obtained by the radiation cross-linking method has high purity and good optical transparency because no additives are required during the cross-linking process.

2.3.2   Preparation of PVA Hydrogel

In the previous study of PVA hydrogel in this study (Trieu & Qutubuddin, 1995), compared with the physical cross-linking method, the mechanical properties of PVA hydrogel obtained by the chemical cross-linking method are one order of magnitude higher, and the resistance of PVA hydrogel. Additionally, the wear performance of the hydrogel is also significantly improved. In the chemical cross-linking method, when the PVA content exceeds 15%, the performance does not change much, and at this time, the molecular chain in the sample is sufficiently cross-linked. In this book, regarding the improved chemical cross-linking method, a PVA hydrogel was prepared according to the research results of the institute. The raw materials for preparing the PVA hydrogel are PVA, DMSO and deionized water, wherein PVA and DMSO are produced by Shanghai Sinopharm Chemical Reagent Co., Ltd. The degree of polymerization of PVA was 1750 ± 50, the degree of alcoholysis was 99.5%, and the concentration of the DMSO solution was >99.0%. PVA is a high molecular polymer, odorless, non-toxic, white or yellowish flocculent, flake or powdery solid with a molecular formula of $(C_2H_4O)n$. DMSO is a colorless and odorless transparent liquid at normal temperature, and is a sulfur-containing organic compound having a molecular formula of $(CH_3)_2SO$. DMSO has the characteristics of hygroscopicity, high polarity, high boiling point and miscibility with water. It has extremely low toxicity and good thermal stability. It is soluble in most organic substances such as ethanol, propanol, benzene and chloroform. DMSO is also used directly in medicine as raw material and carrier for certain drugs. DMSO itself has anti-inflammatory, analgesic, diuretic and sedative effects, and can infiltrate other drugs through skin application.

The specific steps for preparing the PVA hydrogel are as follows: a certain concentration of a mixed solution of DMSO and water is placed at room temperature, generally 80% by weight of DMSO aqueous solution, and a certain amount of PVA is added to the above mixed solution. Heat and stir at 110 °C for about three hours, the PVA is completely dissolved; pour the PVA solution into the prepared stainless steel mold, and then quickly put it into −20 °C for freezing and forming; after a certain period of time, take it out at room temperature and thaw it into pure water. The DMSO component in the sample was completely replaced in the water for one to ten days to obtain a hydrogel sample, which was stored in water at last.

2.4 Structural Observation of Natural Cartilage and Artificial Cartilage

2.4.1 Test Method

The experiment was conducted by using ESEM to observe the surface structure of the surface and section of human articular cartilage, bovine articular cartilage and

PVA hydrogel artificial cartilage, and the elemental composition of the surface. The section and surface particles were measured by an energy spectrometer on the same tester. In the test, the surface of the sample was first observed, the human cartilage and the PVA hydrogel sample were rapidly cooled by liquid nitrogen and the cross-section was broken to observe the cross-section.

Using the preparation method of the natural articular cartilage sample in the above section, the samples of human articular cartilage piece and bovine articular cartilage piece were obtained. The PVA hydrogel was prepared by a modified chemical cross-linking method using 25% by weight and 80% by weight DMSO aqueous solution respectively, the obtained solution had a PVA concentration of 15% by weight, and then was subjected to heating, freezing and thawing operations to obtain two types of observations.

ESEM is a product of Philips (now FEI, USA), model number XL30. SEM is generally used for sample observation. However, it is necessary to fix, dehydrate, and spray gold before the SEM observation, which directly affects the observation of biological materials. ESEM can directly observe the biological sample and retain the moisture in the sample, and can work under three working modes of high vacuum, low vacuum and environment, which is beneficial to observe the original appearance of the sample. Therefore, ESEM is used in this test. The sample is observed. Using the low vacuum mode, the acceleration voltage in the test is 15–20 kV, the size is 4.0–5.0, and the temperature is 4–6 degrees Celsius. In the energy spectrum analysis, the ESEM supporting spectrometer is used, which is the product of the American EDAX company with the model of Genesis.

2.4.2   Observation of Human Cartilage

The result is an ESEM photograph of the surface of human cartilage (see Figure 2-1). It can be seen that the surface of human articular cartilage is flat and non-porous, with a small number of pits and a small number of particles on the surface; there is the presence or absence of a defined layer, and the sample has been frozen and broken by liquid nitrogen that causes the amorphous layer to be picked up. The lower part of the amorphous layer is the cartilage surface layer. It can be seen that there are cell dimples with a diameter of 10 μm or more in the cartilage section, which are cavities filled by chondrocytes, and the porous matrix structure is not observed. Kobayashi (1996) observed the collagen fiber network structure of the cartilage matrix by SEM in the experiment. The porous structure of the matrix was measured to find that the pore diameter was between 0.5 μm and 1 μm. Kobayashi *et al.* performed the operations of drying and spraying gold on the cartilage samples before observation by SEM. The samples were dried when observed, and the liquid phase components in the cartilage were lost, leaving only the porous structure composed of collagen fibers. In this test, ESEM was used as an observation means, and collagen fibers and their porous structures were not found, which may be related to the presence of hydrophilic HA components in the aqueous environment of ESEM and the cartilage structure.

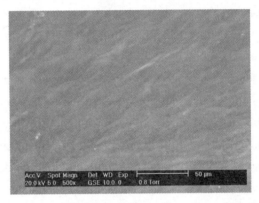

Figure 2-1   ESEM Photographs of the Human Cartilage Surface

2.4.3   Observation of Bovine Cartilage

The result is an ESEM photograph of the surface of bovine cartilage (see Figure 2-2). It can be seen that the surface of bovine articular cartilage is flat without holes or depressions, and there are some particles on the surface; in the smaller cross-section, the cartilage layer, calcification layer and subchondral bone can be seen. The cell lacuna is visible in the cartilage layer. The middle and lower cell lacuna of the cartilage layer are arranged in a certain direction and regularity. The surface layer of the cartilage is irregularly arranged. At the interface between the surface and the interior, the amorphous layer of the surface can be seen. It can be seen from the above results that the surface of bovine articular cartilage is flatter than human articular cartilage; the surface of human articular cartilage and bovine articular cartilage has an amorphous layer, and the existence of lacunar structure and cell lacuna can be seen in the cartilage section. Since ESEM can keep the moisture in the sample from being lost, the collagen fiber network in the two kinds of articular cartilage is difficult to observe.

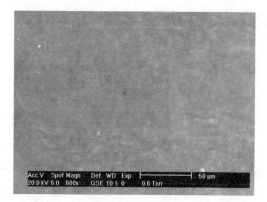

Figure 2-2   ESEM Photographs of Bovine Cartilage Surface

2.4.4   Observation of PVA Hydrogel Artificial Cartilage

(1) PVA hydrogel (80% by weight DMSO)

The result is an ESEM photograph of the surface of a PVA hydrogel (see Figure 2-3). As can be seen from the result, the PVA hydrogel has a smooth surface with some pores of 8–10 microns in diameter; a small amount of internal and surface pores can be seen in the cross-section of the hydrogel near the surface. The result shows an ESEM photograph of a PVA hydrogel section. It can be seen from the cross-sectional view that the PVA hydrogel has a porous structure, the pores are closely arranged, and the pore size varies little; from the magnified view of 2000 times, the pores are closely arranged, and most of the pores have a diameter of about 8 μm.

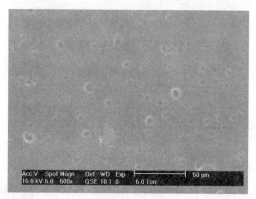

Figure 2-3   ESEM Photographs of PVA Hydrogel Surface

(2) PVA Hydrogel (25% by weight DMSO)

The result is an ESEM photograph of the surface of a PVA hydrogel (see Figure 2-4). It can be seen that the surface of the PVA hydrogel obtained by the 25% by weight aqueous DMSO solution is filled with pores, and most of the pores have a diameter of about 50 μm and a maximum pore diameter of 200 μm. The result shows an ESEM photograph of a PVA hydrogel cross-section. The result shows that the PVA hydrogel has a dense porous structure with a pore size of about 100 microns and irregularities in the shape of the individual pores. From the above results, it can be seen that the PVA hydrogel sample obtained by the 25% by weight aqueous DMSO solution has a larger number and diameter of pores than the sample obtained by the 80% by weight aqueous DMSO solution. The porous structure of the PVA hydrogel obtained by the 80% by weight aqueous DMSO solution is more regular, the shape of the pores is close to a circle, and the internal structure is more compact, which is more favorable for the bearing of the PVA hydrogel. Compared with natural articular cartilage, PVA hydrogel has larger pore sizes, no layered structure similar to cartilage, and no amorphous layer on the surface but holes.

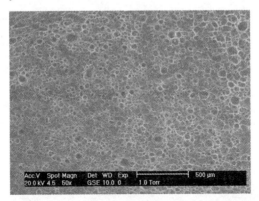

Figure 2-4　ESEM Photographs of PVA Hydrogel Surface

2.4　Analysis of Natural Cartilage Elements

2.4.1　Analysis of Human Cartilage Surface

The picture shows the position of the surface energy spectrum analysis of human cartilage, including Position 1 and Position 2 (see Figure 2-5). It can be seen from the result that the surface particles at Position 1 and the surface at Position 2 contain nitrogen, phosphorus, sulfur and calcium. The surface particles and surface components are basically the same, and strong sulfur appears on the spectrum. Diffraction and phosphorus diffraction peak, which indicates the presence of chondroitin sulfate and phospholipid components on the surface of the cartilage, which is a component of the amorphous layer on the surface of the cartilage. The surface particles contain 0.63% by weight of phosphorus element, 0.52% by weight of sulfur element and 1.07% by weight of calcium element, and the surface contains 0.14% by weight of phosphorus element, 0.39% by weight of sulfur element and 0.28% by weight of calcium element. It is indicated that the surface contains more phosphorus, sulfur and calcium, so the granules may be aggregated from the amorphous layer of the cartilage surface

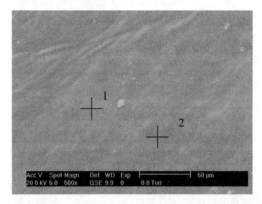

Figure 2-5   EDX Analysis Position of the Human Cartilage Surface

2.4.2   Analysis of Bovine Cartilage Surface

The result shows the positional analysis of the surface energy spectrum of bovine cartilage, including Position 1 and Position 2 (see Figure 2-6). It can be seen from the result that the elemental composition of the surface of the bovine cartilage and the surface particles are identical, and the elemental composition of the particles and the surface indicates that the surface contains chondroitin sulfate and a phospholipid component, wherein the content of the sulfur element in the particle component is 0.64% by weight. The content of the phosphorus element is 0.24% by weight, the content of calcium element is 0.93% by weight, the elemental composition of the particles and the surface are substantially the same, and the calcium element in the particle is slightly higher.

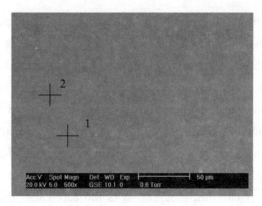

Figure 2-6　EDX Analysis Position of the Bovine Cartilage Surface

Human cartilage has the same elemental composition as the surface and surface particles of bovine cartilage; the content of phosphorus on the surface of bovine cartilage is 0.23% by weight, and the content of sulfur is 0.72% by weight; the content of phosphorus on the surface of human cartilage is 0.14% by weight. The content of the sulfur element is 0.39% by weight; the content of phosphorus element and sulfur element on the surface of human cartilage is slightly lower than that of the bovine cartilage surface, which indicates that the content of chondroitin sulfate and phospholipid in the amorphous layer on the surface of human cartilage is slightly lower.

2.4.3　Sectional Analysis of Cartilage

Bovine articular cartilage was used as the research object in the section elemental analysis of cartilage (see Figure 2-7). In the section of cartilage, among the three positions, the elements of Position 1 and Position 2 have the same composition, and all contain nitrogen, phosphorus and sulfur. The change in elemental content at three different locations is obtained. In Position 1, the content of nitrogen is 14.15% by weight, the content of phosphorus is 0.62% by weight, and the content of sulfur is 1% by weight. In Position 2, the content of nitrogen is 16.69% by weight, the content of phosphorus is 0.25% by weight, and the content of sulfur is 0.95% by weight In Position 1, the content of nitrogen is 16.67% by weight, the content of phosphorus is 0% by weight, and the content of sulfur is 0.73% by weight.

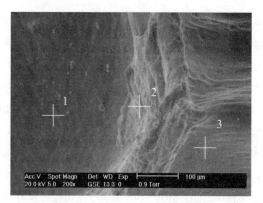

Figure 2-7　EDX Analysis Position of Bovine Cartilage Cross-Section (Left Side Is the Surface)

It can be seen from the result that the phosphorus and sulfur elements in the three positions are gradually decreasing, and the phosphorus content in Position 3 is zero. Position 1 is the surface of the cartilage, and Position 3 is the surface layer of the cartilage (tangential zone), indicating that chondroitin sulfate is present in both the cartilage surface and the surface layer, and the phospholipid component is present only on the surface amorphous layer of cartilage. Studies have shown that phospholipids and HA play an important role in the boundary lubrication of cartilage surfaces (Hills & Buttler, 1984). One of the main phospholipids is dipalmitoyl phosphatidylcholine (DPPC) (Higaki, Murakami, Nakanishi, Miura, Mawatari & Inamoto, 1998; Foy, Iii, Powell, Ishihara, Nakabayashi & LaBerge, 1999). Since phospholipids are only present in the amorphous layer on the surface of cartilage, when the surface of the cartilage is destroyed, it will lack phospholipids as a boundary lubricant for cartilage, and the coefficient of friction of cartilage will rise, which may eventually lead to faster wear of cartilage. In sum, the protection of the amorphous layer on the cartilage surface is necessary.

2.5　Summary

The characteristics of the human joint system and articular cartilage system have been summarized and analyzed, and the histomorphology and biochemical properties of natural articular cartilage are studied; there is also a method of preparing cartilage pin sample and cartilage piece sample that meet the test requirements. Two PVA hydrogel artificial cartilage materials were prepared for testing using an improved chemical cross-linking method.

The surface structure and surface structure of human articular cartilage, bovine articular cartilage and PVA hydrogel artificial cartilage were observed using ESEM. The results showed that the surface of bovine articular cartilage was flatter than the surface of human articular cartilage; the surface of human articular cartilage and bovine articular cartilage had an amorphous layer, and the existence of cell lacuna was observed in the cartilage layer because ESEM maintained the moisture in the sample. It is not lost, so the collagen fiber network in the two articular cartilage is difficult to observe; the PVA hydrogel has a larger pore size than the natural articular cartilage and has no layered structure similar to cartilage, and the surface has pores exposed.

The elemental components of the surface and surface particles of human articular cartilage and bovine articular cartilage were measured, and elemental analysis of the section of bovine cartilage was performed. The results showed that human cartilage had the same elemental composition as the surface and surface particles of bovine cartilage; the content of phosphorus and sulfur on the surface of human cartilage was slightly lower than that of bovine cartilage, indicating that chondroitin sulfate and phospholipid in the amorphous layer of the human cartilage surface. The content of the ingredients was slightly lower; no phosphorus was found in the surface layer of the bovine cartilage, indicating that the phospholipid component only existed on the amorphous layer on the surface of the cartilage.

Chapter 3
Articular Cartilage Surface

3.1 Introduction

In the friction between two solids, the surface condition of the solids directly affects the entire process of friction and wear. Due to the surface roughness, the actual contact between the two surfaces occurs on the discrete microprotrusions. The sum of the contact areas of all microprotrusions is the actual contact area between the two solids, which is only a small fraction of the nominal contact area. When the surface microprotrusions are close, the forces between the atoms cause the microprotrusions to stick and wear during the mutual friction, and the abrasive particles generated by the wear will further damage the surface. For natural cartilage and artificial cartilage, because they are in living organisms, their friction and wear not only affect the lubrication performance of the joint, but also affect the physiological metabolism process. Then it is necessary to study their surface properties.

This chapter systematically studies the surface properties of human cartilage, bovine cartilage and artificial cartilage, obtaines the parameters and changes of surface morphology, surface roughness and surface infiltration, and clarifies the effect of the amorphous layer on the surface of cartilage for the surface properties of cartilage. The relationship between cartilage surface properties and tribological properties is also described.

3.2 Measurement of Surface Roughness of Articular Cartilage

The surface roughness of human articular cartilage, bovine articular cartilage and PVA hydrogel artificial cartilage was measured using a TR100 pocket surface roughness measuring instrument (Beijing Times Group). In the test, the scanning length is 6 mm, and the sampling length is selected to be 0.8 mm. Three horizontal lines and three longitudinal lines on the sheet sample are taken for measurement and averaged. The measurement parameters are the arithmetic mean deviation Ra of the surface contour.

The measurement results of different cartilages are shown in Table 3-1. The roughness values Ra of human cartilage, bovine cartilage, and PVA hydrogel were 2.24 ± 0.39 μm, 1.37 ± 0.37 μm, and 1.47 ± 0.51 μm, respectively. The results showed that the roughness of human cartilage was the largest, and the roughness of bovine cartilage and the roughness of PVA hydrogel were not much different. The roughness of PVA hydrogel was slightly larger than that of bovine cartilage. ESEM observation of cartilage found that the surface of human cartilage was rougher and rougher. The measurement of macroscopic roughness in this experiment was consistent with the results observed in ESEM.

Table 3-1　Surface Roughness of Cartilage

Samples	1	2	3	4	5	6	Average value (in)	Standard deviation (in)
Human cartilage	2.44	2.64	1.78	1.72	2.5	2.35	2.24	0.39
Bovine cartilage	1.45	1.16	1.08	1.18	1.29	2.09	1.37	0.37
PVA hydrogel	1.16	2.04	1.87	1.21	0.73	1.8	1.47	0.51

3.3　AFM-Based Cartilage Surface Study

Atomic force microscope (AFM) was developed based on scanning tunneling microscope (STM). It is imaged by the repulsion gradient information between the probe and the sample. It is not affected by the conductivity of the sample, which makes the sample preparation simple. Compared with traditional microscopy and SEM, AFM can maintain the natural state of the cartilage surface, and can observe the cartilage sample in a liquid environment to avoid the shape change caused by the dry dehydration operation.

3.3.1　Test Method

(1) Sample Preparation

The samples were human articular cartilage, bovine articular cartilage and PVA hydrogel, and the PVA hydrogel was obtained by dissolving 15% PVA in 80% DMSO aqueous solution. Different specimens were fabricated into pin specimens with a diameter of 11 mm to facilitate installation and measurement in the AFM.

(2) Test Equipment and Procedures

The test was carried out using the Nanoscope-III AFM of the American DI Company of Shanghai Jiaotong University. The cantilever beam is triangular (normal elastic coefficient is 0.09 N/m) and the probe tip diameter is about 50 nm. The test temperature is room temperature with humidity of 30%, and the test measurement range is 10×10 μm, sampling number 256, scanning frequency 2 Hz, by AFM liquid observation mode.

3.3.2   AFM Observation of Human Articular Cartilage

The result shows the surface topography of human articular cartilage observed under AFM (see Figure 3-1 before contents). As can be seen from the result, the surface of human cartilage has irregularities and irregularities, and many pits appear. The roughness Ra of human articular cartilage is 68.63 ± 6.22 nm.

3.3.3   AFM Observation of Bovine Articular Cartilage

The result shows the surface topography observed for bovine articular cartilage under AFM (see Figure 3-2 before contents). As can be seen from the result, the surface of bovine cartilage is similar to the surface of human cartilage, the surface is not flat, and many pits appear. The roughness Ra of bovine articular cartilage is 50.16 ± 6.47 nm, and the bovine articular cartilage has a smaller roughness than the roughness of human articular cartilage.

3.3.4   AFM Observation of PVA Hydrogel Artificial Cartilage

The result shows the surface topography observed for PVA hydrogel under AFM (see Figure 3-3 before contents). As can be seen from the result, the surface of the PVA hydrogel is uneven, and the unevenness of the surface of the PVA hydrogel is more regular than that of the human cartilage and bovine cartilage. In the observation of PVA hydrogel by ESEM, it has been found that there are many pores on the surface of the PVA hydrogel, the individual pores are large, and the distribution of these pores can also be observed from the top view of the AFM. The roughness Ra of PVA hydrogel is 59.79 ± 11.13 nm. Compared with human articular cartilage, PVA hydrogel has smaller roughness, but the standard deviation of PVA hydrogel is larger.

The standard deviation of the measured values is relatively large, which is related to the individual large holes on the surface of the PVA hydrogel.

3.4 Effect of the Amorphous Layer on Surface Properties

3.4.1 Surface Observation and Elemental Analysis After Removal of Cartilage Amorphous Layer

In this test, the surface of human cartilage was wiped with a 10% sodium lauryl sulfate solution to remove the amorphous layer on the cartilage surface (see Figure 3-4). A common use of sodium lauryl sulfate is as a denaturant and solubilizing agent for proteins. Almost all proteins can be dissolved in sodium lauryl sulfate, including hydrophobic and denatured proteins (Graindorge, Ferrandez, Ingham, Jin, Twigg & Fisher, 2006).

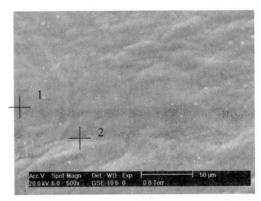

Figure 3-4   ESEM Image of Human Cartilage Without the Amorphous Layer

The result shows an ESEM photograph of the body cartilage after the removal of the amorphous layer on the surface. It can be seen that after the surface amorphous layer is cleaned, the surface of the cartilage becomes very rough, the unevenness of the surface is more obvious, and the particles on the surface of the cartilage are significantly increased. The result shows the results of the analysis of the surface particles of Position 1, and it shows the results of the analysis of the surface of the cartilage of Position 2. As can be seen from the result, both the Position 1 particle and the Position 2 cartilage surface contain nitrogen, sulfur and calcium, and the surface particles and surface components are substantially the same, but the two sites do not contain phosphorus. The result shows that after the test, the phosphorus element has not been added, the sulfur element increased from 0.39% by weight to 1.37% by weight, and the nitrogen element content decreased from 16.12% by weight to 14.35% by weight, indicating that the phospholipid in the surface layer has been completely removed. The increase in sulfur element after the test may be caused by the addition of sulfur in the sodium lauryl sulfate itself. During the cartilage friction process, the phospholipid fraction in the amorphous layer on the cartilage surface is an important lubricant (Forsey, Fisher, Thompson, Stone, Bell & Ingham, 2006). When the amorphous layer on the surface is destroyed and the phospholipid layer disappears, the frictional properties of the cartilage are further reduced.

3.4.2 AFM Observation of Human Articular Cartilage After Removal of the Amorphous Layer

The result shows an AFM observation of the body cartilage after the removal of the amorphous layer on the surface. It can be seen that the height of the human cartilage surface is significantly larger than that of the original state of human cartilage. After the measurement, the roughness of the surface of the human cartilage after removing the amorphous layer on the surface was increased from 68.63 ± 6.22 nm before the test to 72.95 ± 9.79 nm after the test, and the average roughness and standard deviation were significantly increased. It can be seen that the amorphous layer on the surface has a great influence on the surface topography of the cartilage, and the amorphous layer on the surface of the cartilage can make the surface of the cartilage flatter.

3.5 Infiltration Performance of Articular Cartilage Surface

3.5.1 Principle of Contact Angle

The lubricity of the material is related to the wetting property of the surface and the liquid. The better the wettability of the material, the better the lubrication, which reduces the friction and wear of the surface. The wettability of materials and lubricants can be used as an important indicator of the lubricity of materials. Zisman (1964) first studied the polymer material by measuring the contact angle, and further research was carried out by later researchers. Oss & Gilman (1972) used this technique for the determination of biomaterial properties. In reality, the droplets are present on the surface of the material in a relatively stable minimum energy equilibrium state or metastable state, and the apparent contact angle of the lubricating droplets on the surface corresponds to the lowest energy state of the system. The contact angle of a liquid on a solid surface can be defined as a tangential flow through a liquid-gas (or another liquid) interface at the intersection of their three-phase interfaces when the liquid-solid-gas (or another liquid) is in contact. The angle is in the position where it is between solid surfaces. In addition, the interface angle can also be characterized by thermodynamic quantities based on cell adhesion and adsorption. By measuring the contact angle, it is easy to know the degree of hydrophobicity of the substance. The two common conditions in the measurement are shown in the result. It shows that the contact angle is in the range of 90–180 degrees, and the solid surface is not wet. The result shows that the liquid can be fully spread on the solid surface. The larger the contact angle, the more hydrophobic the solid surface is. The small angle indicates that the solid surface is more hydrophilic.

According to the surface thermodynamics, the contact surface is the unit area, and the free energy of the system during the wet process is reduced to

$$-\Delta G = \gamma_{SV} + \gamma_{LV} - \gamma_{SL} = W_A.$$

Among them, γ_{SV}, γ_{LV} and γ_{SL} are the free energy of solid-gas, liquid-gas, and the solid-liquid interface is adhesion work, as shown in the result.

In 1805, Young proposed the equilibrium relationship of the above three-phase junction—Young's equation:

$$\gamma_{SV} - \gamma_{SL} = \gamma_{LV}\cos\theta.$$

θ is the contact angle obtained by

$$W_A = \gamma_{LV}(1 + \cos\theta).$$

From the surface tension and contact angle of the liquid, the adhesion work W_A can be obtained. The adhesion work is the minimum work done by pulling the solid-liquid interface away from the interface. At the $W_A > 0$, the adhesion proceeds automatically, which is the energy criterion for hydrophobicity. At 20 °C, the surface tension of water is 72 mN/m, and the adhesion work can be calculated from the measured contact angle. The contact angle of the commonly used materials is shown in Table 3-2.

Table 3-2　Contact Angles Between Materials and Water

Solid	Contact angle (degree)	Solid	Contact angle (degree)
Paraffin	110	Stainless steel	66
Positive trihexadecane	111	45 steel	68
Polytetrafluoroethylene	107	Al_2O_3	60
Polypropylene	108	Al	76.7
Polyethylene	103	UHMWPE	99

3.5.2　Measurement Method of Contact Angle

According to the geometric characteristics of the sample, the contact angle is tested. The contact angle test method can be divided into a plating method, a capillary method and a powder method. There are three methods for planar solid samples. The first is direct angle measurement. It is an instrument that directly measures the contact angle of the solid-liquid contact interface. Photographic and microscopic methods are commonly used. The second is the droplet size measurement. The droplet size measurement method calculates the contact angle by measuring the droplet size on the solid surface. This method does not require knowledge of the surface tension of the liquid, and its main advantage is that the amount of the sample is small. Commonly used dimensional measurement methods are ellipse method, width and height method, Laplace equation solution and maximum height measurement method. The third type is the optical measurement, which is mainly divided into a specular reflection method and a parallel beam method. The specular reflection method measures the contact angle by specular reflection of the droplets, and the parallel beam method is a further development of the specular reflection method. In addition, there are gravimetric method, filtration pressure method, *etc.* In this test, different samples are measured by the ellipse method and width and height method.

(1) Direct Angle Measurement

The original camera method uses a camera for macro photography or a direct measurement with a microscope with a protractor, but the measurer needs to visually observe the tangential line. Some people have measurement errors, and the resolution of the photo or projection is highly demanded. The current optical contact angle measuring instrument uses a combination of microscope imaging and computer image processing to obtain the contact angle measurement result, which greatly improves the measurement accuracy. Compared with other methods, this method is the most simple and convenient, and the results are more accurate.

(2) Dimensional Measurement

① Ellipse Method

The ellipse method uses an elliptic equation or a trinomial equation to fit the image contour formed by the droplets on the solid surface obtained by the camera to calculate the contact angle value. This method is used in the contact angle measuring instrument. In the elliptical measurement, the baseline is first determined, the contour of the droplet is determined, and the contact angle value is obtained from the contour.

② Width and Height Method

Gravity can be neglected when the droplet is small, and the droplet can be regarded as a part of the ideal sphere, which can be measured by the width and height method. The width and height method measures the droplet height h and the droplet bottom radius r, and determines the contact angle according to the formula. The droplet is considered to be part of a sphere, where R is the diameter of the sphere.

From

$$R = (h^2 + r^2)/2h$$

$$\sin \theta = r/R,$$

so,

$$\sin \theta = 2rh/(h^2 + r^2)$$

$$\tan \frac{\theta}{2} = \frac{h}{r}.$$

When the test is conducted, the forces acting on the water droplets are gravity and adhesion work. Gravity is related to the volume of the liquid. The adhesion work is related to the adhesion area. The contact angle is not dependent on the size of the water droplets. Therefore, there are results:

$$G/W_A \infty^3/r^2 = r.$$

When the radius of the water droplets is enlarged, the influence of gravity is greater. In order to reduce the influence of gravity, the droplets should be minimized (Nakae, Inui, Hirata & Saito, 1998).

For larger droplets, the effect of gravity cannot be completely ignored. The Laplace equation is needed to solve the contour equation of the droplet, as shown in the result. The axisymmetric droplet profile in the gravitational field satisfies:

$$2 + \beta \frac{z}{b} = \frac{1}{R/b} + \frac{\sin \phi}{x/b}$$

$$\beta \equiv b^2 \Delta \rho g / \sigma_{LG}.$$

Ehrlich (1967) solved the differential equation by the perturbation method, which is perfectly applicable to the case where the contact angle is greater than 90 degrees. The solution is to enter the maximum radius of the droplet and the radius of the bottom surface, and the gas surface tension is known.

③ Maximum Height Measurement Method

The specific method of the maximum height measurement method is as follows: the radius of the droplet is r, and the volume is V; when the perturbation occurs, the radius is enlarged and the height is lowered. At the same time, as the solid-liquid phase interface expands $2\pi r \cdot \Delta r$, the gas-liquid and solid-gas interface area also changes to $2\pi r \cdot \Delta r (\gamma_{SL} + \gamma_{LG} - \gamma_{SG})$. The surface free energy of the system increases. At the same time, as the droplet height decreases, the corresponding potential energy decreases to $\frac{1}{2} \rho g V \Delta h$, and the two energy change values are equal:

$$2\pi r \cdot \Delta r (\gamma_{SL} + \gamma_{LG} - \gamma_{SG}) = \frac{1}{2} \rho g V \Delta h.$$

Suppose the droplet is a cylinder and the maximum height of the droplet is h_m,

$$2\pi r \cdot \Delta r h_m = \pi r^2 \cdot \Delta h,$$

so,

$$\gamma_{SL} + \gamma_{LG} - \gamma_{SG} = \frac{1}{2} \rho g h_m^2,$$

substituting Yang's equation

$$\cos \theta' = 1 - \rho g h_m^2 / 2\gamma_L.$$

Among them is the complementary angle of the contact angle; the contact angle is $\theta = \pi - \theta'$; γ_L is the liquid surface tension; ρ is the liquid density, and g is the gravitational acceleration. This method treats the droplet as a cylinder, ignoring the boundary conditions and boundary effects. It requires that it has high requirements for the flatness and size of the measurement surface. When the droplet is no longer increased during the measurement, the measurement liquid needs to be observed by the human eye. There must be a human error; the surface tension, liquid density and gravitational acceleration of the liquid taken in the calculation also have certain errors due to different time and places. Therefore, this method can be used as a comparative reference for other methods, and it is necessary to supplement the method to accurately measure the contact angle.

(3) Optical Measurement—Specular Reflection

Specular reflection was proposed by Langmuir & Schaeffer (1937). The principle is that when a single beam is illuminated onto a three-phase contact line, the observer can see the reflected light in the incident direction of the light when the angle of incidence is equal to the contact angle.

3.5.3　Factors Affecting Contact Angle Measurement

In addition to the influence of contact angle lagging on the measurement results, several aspects have an impact on the measurement.

(1) Effect of Surface Roughness

Wenzel first proposed the effect of solid surface roughness on the contact angle. It is believed that the actual surface has larger surface energy than the ideal surface on the unit surface.

(2) Effects of Surface Adsorption and Surface Contamination

Since the solid and liquid surfaces have a certain adsorption effect on other surrounding media, they have a certain influence on the surface energy.

(3) Gravity

When the volume of the droplet is large, the shape of the droplet is nearly elliptical under the action of gravity, which also affects the measurement result. Take the radius of the droplet as the pressure difference inside and outside the droplet. The gravity effect according to the Laplace formula is

$$\Delta p = \frac{2\gamma_L}{r'}.$$

The volume of liquid used in the test was a few microliters, which was very small, so the effect of gravity was negligible.

(4) The Effect of Temperature and Reading Time

The change in ambient temperature has a certain influence on the measurement. For the measurement system, the contact angle also changes with time, taking relatively stable state readings, and different materials have different time limits.

3.5.4   Test Method

The samples were human articular cartilage, bovine articular cartilage, PVA hydrogel and medical stainless steel. The PVA hydrogel was obtained by dissolving 15% PVA in 80% DMSO aqueous solution. There are five treatment cases of bovine articular cartilage:

(1) The cartilage surface is not treated, and the residual synovial fluid on the surface is evaporated to obtain the sample C1;

(2) The cartilage surface is not treated, and is directly dried at 40 degrees for 3 hours to obtain a sample C2;

(3) The cartilage surface is not treated, and is directly dried at 40 degrees for 8 hours to obtain sample C3;

(4) This step is to use 10% sodium lauryl sulfate solution to scrub the surface of the cartilage to obtain sample C4;

(5) This step is to use 10% sodium lauryl sulfate solution to scrub the surface of the cartilage, with vacuum drying at 40 degrees for 8 hours to obtain sample C5.

For the C1 and C2 samples, in order to prevent the influence of residual synovial fluid on the surface to obtain a relatively stable contact angle, the cartilage was allowed to stand at room temperature for 1.5 hours, and the contact angle measurement was performed after the surface liquid was completely evaporated.

Human articular cartilage pieces were prepared and treated accordingly as a comparison with bovine articular cartilage:

(1) The cartilage surface is not treated, and the residual synovial fluid on the surface is evaporated to obtain the sample RC1;

(2) This step is to scrub the surface of the cartilage with a 10% sodium lauryl sulfate solution to obtain a sample RC4.

PVA hydrogel samples are divided into 3 cases:

(1) This step is to leave no residual moisture on the surface of the sample at room temperature to obtain sample P1;

(2) The hydrogel is dried under vacuum at 40 degrees for 3 hours to obtain a sample P2;

(3) The hydrogel is dried under vacuum at 40 degrees for 8 hours to obtain a sample P3.

Stainless steel is medical stainless steel 317L, roughness Ra is 0.05 microns, and sample code is S1. The test was carried out using the OCA-20 optical contact angle measuring instrument of the German Dataphysics Company of the Analysis and Testing Center of Shanghai Jiao Tong University. The liquid was used for measurement, and the test liquid was used for physiological saline to measure the ambient temperature. Each sample was measured 6 times and the results were averaged.

3.5.5   Contact Angles of Different Materials

The results can be seen in Table 3-3, Table 3-4 and Table 3-5.

Table 3-3   Contact Angles of Bovine Cartilage

Sample	Method	Test 1	Test 2	Test 3	Test 4	Test 5	Test 6	Mean	SD
C1	Ellipse method	84	90.2	95.2	95.4	96.4	88.2	91.6	4.9
	Width and height method	82.8	88.6	92	91.3	94.9	87.2	89.5	4.2
C2	Ellipse method	80.5	81.7	88.5	86.1	90.1	90.7	86.3	4.3
	Width and height method	78.4	80.9	81.5	82.3	89.2	88	83.4	4.3
C3	Ellipse method	73.4	76.1	76.4	82.5	83.4	74.5	77.7	4.2
	Width and height method	71.1	73.9	74.3	79.4	78.6	74.2	75.3	3.1
C4	Ellipse method	29.5	38.7	39.8	33.4	32.2	31.4	34.2	4.1
	Width and height method	31.6	36.3	34.4	28.2	32.1	33.1	32.6	2.7
C5	Ellipse method	75.7	60.2	65.1	61.8	67.4	59.1	64.9	6.1
	Width and height method	72.8	59.7	62.9	58.2	65.3	60.6	63.3	5.3

Table 3-4   Contact Angles of Stainless Steel and Human Cartilage

Sample	Method	Test 1	Test 2	Test 3	Test 4	Test 5	Test 6	Mean	SD
S1	Ellipse method	72.7	64.9	61.6	60.9	62.8	70.3	65.5	4.9
	Width and height method	67.6	63.2	59.2	57.7	59.8	68.7	62.7	4.6

(to be continued)

Sample	Method	Test 1	Test 2	Test 3	Test 4	Test 5	Test 6	Mean	SD
RC1	Ellipse method	80.1	80.6	85.1	87.8	87.4	81.7	83.8	3.4
	Width and height method	78.2	77.8	83.5	86.2	85.8	79.6	81.9	3.8
RC4	Ellipse method	29.2	29.5	33.5	35.9	30.4	36.4	32.5	3.2
	Width and height method	28.1	28.5	31.2	34	33.5	35.1	31.7	2.9

Table 3-5　Contact Angles of PVA Hydrogel

Sample	Method	Test 1	Test 2	Test 3	Test 4	Test 5	Test 6	Mean	SD
P1	Ellipse method	20.6	22.2	18.8	17.9	10.4	11.9	17	4.8
	Width and height method	18.6	20.9	16.9	14.2	11.4	12.7	15.8	3.6
P2	Ellipse method	28	33.1	32.2	30.3	33.9	26.1	30.6	3.1
	Width and height method	27.6	30.7	29.7	26.3	28.7	24.4	27.9	2.3
P3	Ellipse method	69.7	68.8	69.2	75.4	75.6	74.8	72.3	3.3
	Width and height method	67.8	68.7	67.4	74.1	75.1	73.4	71.1	3.5

(1) Comparison of Ellipse Method and Width and Height Method

It can be seen that the result of the bovine cartilage C1 obtained by the ellipse method is 91.6 ± 4.9 degrees, and the result of the width and height method is 89.5 ± 4.2 degrees. It can be seen that the results of the two measurement methods are not much different, and the results obtained by the width and height method are slightly less than the result of the ellipse method.

During the test, although the droplets are already small, the gravity of the droplets still has a certain influence on the measurement results. In the formula of the dimension measurement method, after the droplet is dropped on the surface of the sample, it is not ideally spherical under the action of gravity, and the height is smaller than the height of the ideal sphere. When the contact angle is large, the influence of gravity is more significant, so the formula is calculated. The contact angle is smaller than the ideal state. Since the overall trend of the results obtained by the two methods is consistent, the following analysis discusses the results obtained by the elliptic method.

(2) Contact Angles of Different Materials

The result shows the contact angles of cartilage, artificial cartilage and stainless steel before and after the sodium lauryl sulfate scrub test in the original wet state (see Figure 3-5). As can be seen from the result, the contact angle of bovine cartilage is 91.6 ± 4.9 degrees, the contact angle of human cartilage is 83.8 ± 3.4 degrees, the contact angle of hydrogel is 17 ± 4.8 degrees, and the stainless steel 317 L is 65.5 ± 4.9 degrees. The contact angle of the gel is smaller than that of natural cartilage, that is, the infiltration performance of the hydrogel is better than that of natural cartilage. The stainless steel 317 L is only smaller than the value of cartilage; the contact angle of bovine cartilage is larger than the contact angle of human cartilage, and the infiltration performance of human cartilage is superior to that of bovine cartilage.

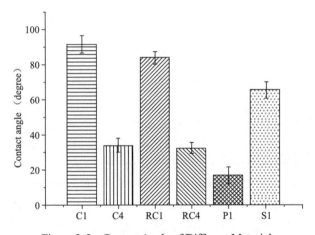

Figure 3-5　Contact Angle of Different Materials

In addition, it can be found that the contact angle of cartilage and cartilage in the original wet state is quite different. The contact angle of bovine cartilage changes from 91.6 ± 4.9 degrees at the beginning to 34.2 ± 4 degrees after scrubbing, and the contact angle of human cartilage, from 83.8 ± 3.4 degrees in the beginning to 32.5 ± 3.2 degrees after scrubbing. The 10% sodium lauryl sulfate solution in this test can effectively remove the amorphous layer on the cartilage surface, so that the surface of the cartilage no longer has the protection of the amorphous layer and the droplet can directly contact the porous structure of the cartilage. The contact angle becomes small and the wettability is improved.

(3) The Contact Angle of Cartilage and Artificial Cartilage Varies with Drying Time

The result shows the changes in bovine cartilage and hydrogel as a function of drying time. As the drying time reaches 8 hours, the contact angle of bovine cartilage is reduced from 91.6 ± 4.9 degrees to 77.7 ± 4.2 degrees. The contact angle of the hydrogel during drying increased from 17 ± 4.8 degrees to 72.3 ± 3.3 degrees. In the beginning, the contact angle of the hydrogel is much smaller than the contact angle of the cartilage. As the drying time increases, the contact angle values of the two gradually approach. As the drying time is extended to 8 hours, the change in the contact angle of the cartilage is moderated than the change in the hydrogel, and is maintained above 70 degrees.

The amorphous layer above the tangential layer of the cartilage surface contains glycoproteins (Orford & Gardner, 1985), chondroitin, keratan sulfate, proteoglycans (Kobayashi, Yonekubo & Kurogouchi, 1995), phospholipids (Hills, 1989), polymers of HA, proteins and so on. The amorphous layer on the surface can effectively reduce the permeability of the cartilage surface. When the droplets are dripped on the surface of the cartilage, the layer is in contact with the droplets to make the cartilage hydrophobic, so the wettability of the surface of the fresh cartilage is poor. When the cartilage is dried at 40 degrees for 3 hours or 8 hours, the amorphous layer on the surface is destroyed by drying, the moisture content of the cartilage itself is also largely evaporated, and the cartilage table begins to deform, as found by Crockett, Roos, Rossbach, Dora, Born & Troxler (2005) by ESEM. Later, deformation and wrinkles appear on the dehydrated surface, as shown in the result. The loss of the amorphous layer on the cartilage surface, as well as the grooves formed by the shrinkage deformation, make the liquid easier to spread, causing a reduction in the surface contact angle.

Although the internal structure of the hydrogel is similar to the porous structure of cartilage, the surface layer has no structure similar to the amorphous layer. When the droplet drops onto the surface of the hydrogel, it directly contacts the porous structure, and the liquid is more easily spread out, so the water is condensed. The infiltration of the glue is better. When the hydrogel is dried at 40 degrees for 3 hours or 8 hours, the water in the porous structure of the hydrogel is continuously lost, the solid skeleton of the hydrogel gradually shrinks, and the voids in the skeleton are simultaneously reduced, resulting in a decrease in the wetting property. The contact angle gradually becomes larger.

(4) Changes in Cartilage Contact Angle with Drying Time After Sodium Lauryl Sulfate Scrubbing

The result shows the change in the contact angle of bovine cartilage with drying time. After 40 hours or 8 hours of drying, the contact angle of bovine cartilage in the original state was reduced from 91.6 ± 4.9 degrees to 77.7 ± 4.2 degrees, and the contact angle of bovine cartilage increased from 34.2 ± 4 degrees to 64.9 ± 6.1 degrees after scrubbing. The contact angle of bovine cartilage is reduced, and the cartilage is increased after scrubbing. After 8 hours of drying, the cartilage infiltration after scrubbing was further reduced, similar to the change in the hydrogel after drying. During the long-term drying process, although the cause of the destruction of the amorphous layer is different, the amorphous layer on the surface of the cartilage after cartilage and scrubbing is gradually destroyed, and the contact angle values of the two begin to approach each other.

3.5.6　Surface Tension and Adhesion Work

At the interface of the two-phase system, the state of the substance molecules is different from the state of the molecules inside the phases. When there is an examination inside the object, the force of the molecules surrounding each molecule is symmetrical, the forces cancel each other out, and their resultant force is equal to zero. However, the molecules in the surface layer are different. On the one hand, they are affected by the internal molecules of the phase. On the other hand, by the molecules in the other phase of different properties, the surface area of the surface layer is the same as the area dispersed inside the phase. There is residual energy compared to the upper one. This residual energy is called surface tension on the surface of the liquid and surface free energy on the solid surface. When the surface tension of the liquid is equal to or lower than the free energy of the surface of the material, the liquid can spread over the surface of the material.

γ_{SV}, γ_{LV} and γ_{SL} are related (Chappuis, Sherman, Neumann, 1983; Neumann, Absolom, Francis & Oss, 1980),

$$\gamma_{SL} = \frac{\left(\sqrt{\gamma_{SV}} - \sqrt{\gamma_{LV}} \right)^2}{1 - 0.015 \sqrt{\gamma_{SV}\gamma_{LV}}},$$

then $\gamma_{SV} - \gamma_{SL} = \gamma_{LV}\cos\theta$, so

$$\cos\theta = \frac{(0.015\gamma_{SV} - 2)\sqrt{\gamma_{SV} + \gamma_{LV}} + \gamma_{LV}}{\gamma_{LV}(0.015\sqrt{\gamma_{SV}\gamma_{LV}} - 1)}.$$

The surface tension of saline is $\gamma_{LV} = 72.5$ mN/m, adhesion work is got by the formula $W_A = \gamma_{LV}(1 + \cos\theta)$. The surface free energy of the C1 sample is 27.6 mN/m, and the adhesion work is 70.5 mN/m. The results can be seen in Table 3-6.

Table 3-6 Surface Free Energy and Adhesive Work

Sample	C1	C2	C3	C4	C5	P1	P2	P3	RC1	RC4	S1
Surface free energy γ_{SV} (mN/m)	27.6	31.3	36.4	62	44.1	69.5	63.5	40	32.6	62.5	43.6
Adhesion work W (mN/m)	70.5	77.2	87.9	132.5	103.3	141.8	134.9	94.5	80.3	133.6	102.6

3.6 Analysis of the Influence of Surface Properties of the Articular Cartilage on Friction Performance

3.6.1 Effect of the Surface Amorphous Layer on Friction Properties

In the experiment, the surface of human cartilage was wiped with 10% sodium lauryl sulfate solution to remove the amorphous layer on the cartilage surface. After washing, the surface of the cartilage became very rough. It can be seen that the unevenness of the surface was more obvious, and the surface of the cartilage surface increased significantly. The phosphorus element was not detected, the sulfur element increased from 0.39% by weight to 1.37% by weight, and the nitrogen element content decreased from 16.12% by weight to 14.35% by weight. When using AFM to examine the samples, the surface roughness of human cartilage was significantly increased, and the roughness increased from 68.63 ± 6.22 nm before the test to 72.95 ± 9.79 nm after the test. The average roughness and standard deviation of the roughness increased significantly. In the frictional motion of the cartilage and the artificial joint material, the cartilage contacts the other material through the surface and generates friction. On the one hand, the amorphous layer on the surface can protect the internal structure of the cartilage from damage. On the other hand, the intrinsic component of the amorphous layer on the surface, especially the phospholipid component, can be used as a boundary lubricant to reduce friction.

After the cartilage loses its amorphous surface, the surface becomes rougher and the depression is more pronounced, which also increases the friction during movement. It can be seen that protecting the amorphous layer of the cartilage surface is crucial to ensure good tribological performance of the cartilage.

3.6.2   Effect of Wetting Properties on Friction Properties

Natural articular cartilage plays a role in cushioning and lubricating in the human body. The purpose of developing artificial cartilage such as hydrogel is to replace or partially replace damaged natural cartilage, which requires improving the lubrication performance of artificial cartilage. The range of motion of the joint is low-speed heavy load, and most of the time is in the boundary lubrication state, which has high requirements on the friction performance of cartilage and artificial cartilage, and the lubricating properties of cartilage. So, artificial cartilage is closely related to its infiltration performance. Chappuis, Sherman & Neumann (1983) proposed the principle of non-wetting lubrication of joints to explain the friction properties of articular cartilage. As shown in the result, for a homogenous horizontal plane of two distances, when a drop of liquid is placed between them, the force exerted by the droplet on the plane can be expressed as

$$F = \frac{\pi \gamma_{LV} r}{h}(-\cos \theta_A - \cos \theta_B) - 2\pi r \gamma_{LV} \sin \theta_B.$$

r is the droplet radius;

γ_{LV} is the surface tension of the liquid;

h is the distance between the two planes;

θ_A and θ_B are the contact angles of the liquid to the plane.

3.7   Summary

The roughness of human cartilage, bovine articular cartilage and PVA hydrogel artificial cartilage was measured by surface roughness measuring instrument. The results showed that the roughness of human cartilage was larger than the roughness of bovine cartilage and the roughness of PVA hydrogel. The degree of difference is not large, and the roughness of PVA hydrogel is slightly larger than that of bovine cartilage.

AFM was used to observe the surface of human articular cartilage, bovine articular cartilage and PVA hydrogel artificial cartilage, and the micro-roughness was measured. The roughness Ra of human articular cartilage was 68.63 ± 6.22 nm, and the roughness Ra of bovine articular cartilage obtained was 50.16 ± 6.47 nm. The roughness Ra of the PVA hydrogel was 59.79 ± 11.13 nm. The surface of cartilage and PVA hydrogel was observed by AFM. It was found that the surface of bovine cartilage was similar to that of human cartilage, and many pits appeared on the surface. Bovine articular cartilage had smaller micro-roughness than human articular cartilage. The microscopic roughness of the PVA hydrogel was between human cartilage and bovine cartilage, but the standard deviation of the measured values obtained was relatively large.

The amorphous layer on the cartilage surface has an important influence on its friction properties. After the surface of the human cartilage is wiped to remove the amorphous layer on the surface of the cartilage, the surface of the cartilage becomes very rough. The unevenness of the surface is more obvious, and the particles on the surface of the cartilage are significantly increased. The surface roughness of cartilage increased from 68.63 ± 6.22 nm before the test to 72.95 ± 9.79 nm after the test, and the average roughness and standard deviation increased significantly. In the frictional motion of the cartilage and the artificial joint material, the cartilage contacts the other material through the surface and generates friction. On the one hand, the amorphous layer on the surface can protect the internal structure of the cartilage from damage. On the other hand, the intrinsic component of the amorphous layer on the surface, especially the phospholipid component, can be used as a boundary lubricant to reduce the friction between the friction pairs. At the same time, after the cartilage loses its amorphous layer on the surface, the surface becomes rougher and the depression is more pronounced, which also increases the friction during exercise. It can be seen that protecting the amorphous layer of the cartilage surface is crucial to ensure the good tribological performance of the cartilage.

The contact angles of human cartilage, bovine cartilage, PVA hydrogel, and medical stainless steel 317 L were measured with physiological saline. The contact angle of bovine cartilage was 91.6 ± 4.9 degrees, the contact angle of human cartilage was 83.8 ± 3.4 degrees, the contact angle of hydrogel was 17 ± 4.8 degrees, and the stainless steel 317 L was 65.5 ± 4.9 degrees; the contact angle of hydrogel was less than natural cartilage. The stainless steel 317 L is only smaller than the value of cartilage; the contact angle of bovine cartilage is greater than the contact angle of human cartilage. The contact angle of the cartilage in the original wet state and the cartilage after removing the amorphous layer on the surface is quite different: the contact angle of bovine cartilage changes from 91.6 ± 4.9 degrees at the beginning to 34.2 ± 4 degrees after scrubbing. The contact angle of human cartilage changed from 83.8 ± 3.4 degrees at the beginning to 32.5 ± 3.2 degrees after scrubbing. With a drying time of 8 hours, the contact angle of bovine cartilage decreased from 91.6 ± 4.9 degrees to 77.7 ± 4.2 degrees. The contact angle of the hydrogel during drying increased from 17 ± 4.8 degrees to 72.3 ± 3.3 degrees. As the drying time was extended to 8 hours, the change in the contact angle of the cartilage was less moderated than the change in the hydrogel, and was maintained above 70 degrees.

The infiltration performance of the cartilage surface has an important influence on its friction performance. The higher contact angle of the cartilage surface facilitates the retention of synovial fluid for non-wetting lubrication. Moreover, the cartilage surface also has a large number of depressions, which also contributes to the maintenance of the lubricating liquid. After the cartilage is deformed by pressure, the liquid contained in the cartilage also oozes out to act as a lubricating fluid. After the amorphous layer is removed, the contact angle of the cartilage is significantly reduced, which is not conducive to the maintenance of the lubricating fluid on the surface of the cartilage friction and leads to an increase in the contact of the cartilage solid phase, thus causing an increase in friction. The PVA hydrogel has a small contact angle, which reduces the ability of the lubricating fluid to carry on the two friction surfaces and is not conducive to reducing the friction of the joint surface. The further improvement of the PVA hydrogel can be achieved by improving the surface properties by the multi-layered bionic design of the PVA hydrogel, including adding an amorphous layer rich in boundary lubricant to the surface by various attachment means, improving the performance of the internal porous structure, and reducing or eliminating the surface of the hole exposed.

Chapter 4
Mechanical Properties of the Articular Cartilage Surface and Exposure Studies

4.1 Introduction

The components of articular cartilage account for 80% of the total weight and the rest are matrix components. Type II collagen fibers and proteoglycans in articular cartilage are interlaced to form a network structure to carry body weight (Mow & Lai, 1980). When the articular cartilage moves to each other, the fluid flow in the cartilage is resisted and cannot flow freely in the matrix network structure, and the macroscopic performance is the mechanical properties of the cartilage. When OA or accidental injury occurs, the articular cartilage will be destroyed and lose its original function. For example, when OA occurs, the tensile mechanical properties of the affected knee cartilage will be significantly smaller than normal knee articular cartilage, which directly affects the motor function and tribological properties of cartilage. In order to restore the normal function of the joint, it is necessary to replace the damaged joint with an artificial joint. Traditional artificial joint materials have been improved for decades and their service life is still difficult to achieve, so many new artificial cartilage materials have been studied and applied (Covert, Ott & Ku, 2003). As a new type of artificial cartilage material, PVA hydrogel has a porous structure similar to natural cartilage, can maintain a large amount of water, has good biocompatibility, can be used to replace diseased cartilage, and is also used as the artificial nucleus or drug carrier. In order to achieve the purpose of replacing the diseased cartilage and restoring joint function, higher requirements are put forward for the mechanical properties of PVA hydrogel. At present, the research on the biomechanical properties of knee joint cartilage is mainly based on the stretching of cartilage, and the lack of mechanical properties of natural cartilage and artificial cartilage. In this chapter, the compression properties of natural articular cartilage and PVA hydrogel artificial cartilage are compared. Compressive stress-strain, stress relaxation and creep tests are performed respectively. The stress-strain and time of articular cartilage and PVA hydrogel artificial cartilage are obtained. Relationship and analysis of the biomechanical properties of articular cartilage are studied.

Artificial joint materials commonly used in clinical practice include cobalt-chromium molybdenum alloy, UHMWPE and ceramics, *etc.*, which are hard materials. One of the key factors determining the frictional condition of cartilage and artificial joint material is the surface contact state of the cartilage with the artificial joint material. At present, there are no effective means to directly observe their surface contact conditions. Therefore, in this chapter, glass, which is also a hard material, is used as an alternative to observe the surface contact state of cartilage and glass.

4.2 Mechanical Properties Test of Articular Cartilage

4.2.1 Test Method

(1) Sample Preparation

Using the sample processing method in previous documents, the obtained samples were human articular cartilage, bovine articular cartilage and PVA hydrogel, and the PVA hydrogel was obtained by dissolving 15% PVA in 80% DMSO aqueous solution.

The special stainless steel circular cutter with an inner diameter of 4.5 mm was prepared for cutting the sample. The surface of the cartilage piece was observed with a naked eye and a stereo microscope, a smooth and non-destructive cartilage surface was selected, and then a circular cartilage sample was cut perpendicular to the joint surface with a special knife to obtain a sample having a diameter of 4.5 mm and a thickness of 1.6-1.9 mm. The PVA hydrogel sample was used, a 4.5 mm diameter hydrogel sample was cut with a special knife and the sample thickness was about 1.7 mm. Each test used 6 samples in each case.

(2) Test Equipment

The compression test equipment is the UMT-3 multi-micro friction wear tester of CETR Company of the United States. The testing machine can realize accurate dynamic loading through the closed-loop servo system. The force can be as small as 0.1 mN and the minimum moving speed is 0.001 mm/s. Micro-tribological and mechanical properties testing of various materials and lubricants enables simultaneous in-situ measurements of multiple signals such as load, friction, torque, contact resistance, and longitudinal displacement. In the test, the cartilage was first tested for compressive strength, and a reasonable stress level was determined according to the results, followed by creep and relaxation tests. The compression device is shown in the result. The upper 12 mm diameter stainless steel round indenter is combined with the lower diameter 40 mm stainless steel circular platform for compression test. The upper stainless steel circular indenter is connected to the force sensor through the indenter clamp (see Figure 4-1).

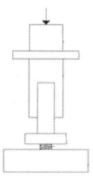

Figure 4-1   The Compression Test Device

(3) Test Procedures

Modulus measurement of articular cartilage materials was currently regulated without standards. The test was carried out with reference to the test methods and procedures in GB/T1041-92. Before the test, the caliper first accurately measured the original thickness of the cartilage or hydrogel sample and averaged it to calculate the strain rate. Then it adjusted the testing machine, and placed the sample between the two platens. The sample centerline coincided with the centerline of the two platen surfaces to ensure that the end face of the specimen was parallel to the surface of the platen. The surface of the platen was just in contact with the end face of the sample, and the zero point of the deformation was determined. In the compressive stress-strain test, the compression speed was 0.01 mm/s (0.6 mm/min). During the compression process, the testing machine came with software to record the axial load and axial displacement of the applied force in real-time. In the creep test, the load was kept constant at 15 N (0.94 MPa), and the change in strain of the sample was measured in 6 minutes. In the stress relaxation test, the sample was kept at a strain state of 30%, and the change in the stress of the sample within 6 minutes was recorded. The results of the creep test and the stress relaxation test was fitted using a function.

4.2.2　Stress-Strain Relationship of Cartilage

The result shows the comparison of the stress-strain relationship of human cartilage, bovine cartilage, and PVA hydrogel artificial cartilage (see Figure 4-2).

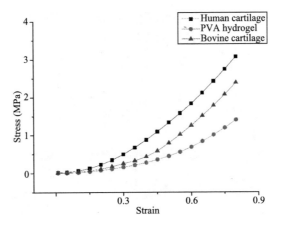

Figure 4-2　The Stress-Strain Relationship Curves

Both cartilage and PVA hydrogel are viscoelastic materials. Compressive deformation occurs after the force is applied. The stress-strain curve reflects the deformation ability of different materials under stress. The larger the deformation, the stronger the viscosity and the weaker the elasticity. As can be seen in Figure 4-2 trend curves, cartilage and PVA hydrogel continuously increase large stress, and gradually increase the degree of deformation; PVA degree of deformation of the hydrogel is greater than the human cartilage and bovine cartilage. Moreover, the PVA hydrogel has less elasticity. The data curve of stress and strain is fitted and compared by exponential growth function called Exponential Growth 1. The function expression formula is

$$y = y_0 + A_1 e^{x/t_1}. \tag{4-1}$$

Among them, A_1 is the intensity, and t_1 is the growth range. The values of the obtained function parameters are shown in Table 4-1.

Table 4-1   The Fit Parameters of Stress-Strain Relationship

Sample	Fitting parameter		
	y_0	A_1	t_1
Human articular cartilage	-0.23133 ± 0.05233	0.2325 ± 0.04951	0.2895 ± 0.02444
Bovine articular cartilage	-0.12045 ± 0.0127	0.11529 ± 0.0104	0.25366 ± 0.00871
PVA hydrogel	-0.03951 ± 0.01103	0.04329 ± 0.01063	0.22161 ± 0.017

4.2.3   Compression Modulus of Cartilage

The strain value of 75% was calculated stress and strain values obtained at the compressive modulus have been known compression modulus:

$$E' = \frac{\sigma}{\varepsilon},$$
(4-2)

where E'—compression modulus, unit MPa;

σ—any stress value in the linear range of the stress-strain curve, in units of MPa;

ε—the strain value corresponding to the stress in the linear range of the stress-strain curve.

At the same time, the relationship between the elastic modulus and the compressive modulus is as follows, where v is the Poisson's ratio:

$$E' = \frac{(1 - v)E}{(1 + v)(1 - 2v)}.$$

Get $$E' = \frac{(1 - v)E}{(1 + v)(1 - 2v)}.$$
(4-3)

According to Formula (4-2), the compression modulus of human articular cartilage is 3.6492 ± 0.6199 MPa, the compression modulus of PVA hydrogel is 1.5951 ± 0.1469 MPa, and the compression modulus of bovine articular cartilage is 2.7645 ± 0.3667 MPa. It can be seen that the compression modulus of articular cartilage is greater than the compression modulus of PVA hydrogel and bovine articular cartilage, and the compression modulus of PVA hydrogel is the smallest. The Poisson's ratio of human and bovine lateral ankle cartilage was 0.1 and 0.4, respectively (Ateshian & Hung, 2006). According to Formula (4-3), the elastic modulus of human articular cartilage was $3.5681 \pm 0. 6061$ MPa, and the elastic modulus of bovine articular cartilage was 1.2901 ± 0.1711 MPa.

4.2.4 Cartilage Creep

The result is the creep curve of human cartilage, bovine cartilage, and PVA hydrogel artificial cartilage (see Figure 4-3).

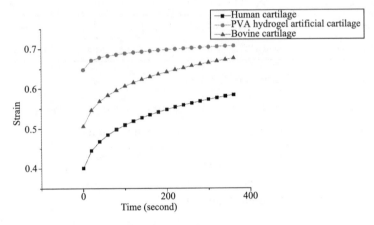

Figure 4-3   The Creep Curve

In the creep test, the sample is compressed and loaded to a certain load, the load applied to the sample is kept constant, and the sample continues to deform. It is observed that the change in the amount of deformation of the sample needs a certain period of time. The exponential growth curve fit function (Exponential Growth 1) is used and fit, and the function obtained parameter values are shown in Table 4-2.

Table 4-2   The Fit Parameter of Creep Curves

Sample	Fitting parameter		
	Y_0	A_1	T_1
Human articular cartilage	0.58874 ± 0.00461	-0.17638 ± 0.00465	-127.57563 ± 9.99703
Bovine articular cartilage	0.68054 ± 0.00438	-0.16379 ± 0.0044	-128.34745 ± 10.24716
PVA hydrogel artificial cartilage	0.70455 ± 0.00156	-0.05055 ± 0.00265	-81.98725 ± 10.61583

4.2.5 Stress Relaxation of Cartilage

The result is a stress relaxation curve of human cartilage, bovine cartilage, and PVA hydrogel artificial cartilage (see Figure 4-4).

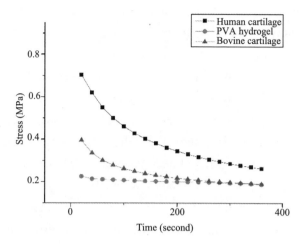

Figure 4-4　The Stress Relaxation Curves

In the stress relaxation test, the sample is compressed and loaded to a certain deformation, the amount of compression of the sample is kept constant, the pressure change of the sample to the compression member is observed for a certain period of time, and the change of the pressure is converted into a stress change. The obtained curve is fitted using an exponential growth fit function (Exponential Growth 1), and the obtained function parameter values are shown in Table 4-3.

Table 4-3　The Fit Parameters of Stress Relaxation Curves

Sample	Fitting parameter		
	Y0	A1	T1
Human articular cartilage	0.25127 ± 0.00501	0.52871 ± 0.00665	−110.82907 ± 3.99893
Bovine articular cartilage	0.19339 ± 0.00268	0.24735 ± 0.00699	−79.24299 ± 4.51634
PVA hydrogel	0.1866 ± 0.00444	0.0379 ± 0.00339	−184.08778 ± 53.02671

4.3　Analysis of the Effect of Mechanical Properties of the Articular Cartilage on Friction Performance

The excellent tribological properties of articular cartilage are directly related to its biomechanical properties, and articular cartilage damage is also the result of decreased biomechanical properties. In this test, the elasticity of human articular cartilage was measured to be greater than that of bovine articular cartilage and PVA hydrogel. In the same stress state under the condition, the strain value of PVA hydrogel bovine articular cartilage is greater than the minimum strain values human articular cartilage. The compression modulus of articular cartilage was calculated to be the largest, followed by bovine articular cartilage, and the compression modulus of PVA hydrogel was the smallest. Articular cartilage plays a role in the body's weight and maintains the joint's low friction. PVA hydrogel, as a cartilage substitute material, also needs to evaluate its performance according to similar working conditions. In articular cartilage, collagen fibers and proteoglycans aggregate to form a porous network structure. It is shown that the proteoglycan contained therein is very hydrophilic. The PVA hydrogel also has a three-dimensional porous network similar to cartilage and does not delaminate itself. The porous structure of the cartilage is denser than that of the PVA hydrogel, and the cartilage itself has a layered structure. This makes the cartilage better than the PVA hydrogel from the bearing capacity to its friction performance. It can be seen from the test results that the ability of the articular cartilage to carry pressure against deformation during continuous compression is superior to PVA hydrogel. The presence of hydrophilic proteoglycans and collagen fibers in the cartilage promotes the cartilage bearing pressure, and the cartilage mechanical properties are better when the collagen fiber content is large (Byers, Moore, Byard & Fazzalari, 2000; Wachtel, Maroudas & Schneiderman, 1995).

In the creep test and the stress relaxation test, the degree of change in stress or strain of the two materials can be seen. In the creep test, the strain of human cartilage changed more than the initial strain value of the PVA hydrogel, and the stress of the human cartilage in the stress relaxation test also changed from the initial value to the PVA hydrogel. The change of bovine cartilage was between human cartilage and PVA hydrogel. It can be seen from the stress-strain test results that the deformation of human cartilage under the same stress state is smaller than that of PVA hydrogel, and the stress of human cartilage under the same strain condition is greater than that of PVA hydrogel.

There is a study on the mechanical properties of the cartilage. Mow, Kuei, Lai & Armstrong (1980) used the basic equations of continuum mechanics, and constitutive equations derived articular cartilage is referred to as two-phase theory (Biphasic Theory). The theory is that the cartilage can be seen as a solid and a liquid phase and regarded as a combination of phases. With the force of the articular cartilage, the water in the liquid phase carries a certain load and flows continuously in the solid matrix. The solid phase, that is, the solid matrix, is mainly composed of collagen fibers and proteoglycans, and is also subjected to a certain load. Articular cartilage contains approximately 80% water. At the beginning of the fixed load, the water in the articular cartilage bears the main load, but as time goes on, the water is continuously lost and the load is transferred to the solid phase matrix. In the case where the stress on the cartilage remains unchanged, as the liquid phase is lost, the solid phase matrix is subjected to an increasingly large load and the strain rapidly becomes large. In the case where the strain of the cartilage remains unchanged, the loss of the liquid phase causes a continuous decrease in the cartilage stress. It is found that 15% of the PVA hydrogel contains about 60.3% water. The water content of the PVA hydrogel is less than articular cartilage. At the beginning of the test, the solid substrate has a large load carrier, and the load kept constant in the process. So, the load transmitted from the liquid phase to the solid phase is less, the hydrogel creeps and the relaxation amount is smaller than the human articular cartilage.

With the growth of age, proteoglycans in aged or arthritic cartilage are significantly reduced (Hardingham & Bayliss, 1991), which alters the ability of the cartilage to retain moisture and accelerates the flow of the liquid phase. Thus, tests showed that it reduces the liquid phase load and increases the solids. The bearing of the phase matrix increases the friction of the cartilage during the movement of the human body, resulting in damage to the cartilage. For artificial cartilage, increasing the liquid phase content and increasing its load-carrying capacity can effectively reduce the possibility of damage.

It can be seen from the test results that in order to make the artificial cartilage closer to the natural cartilage, it is necessary to improve the mechanical properties of the PVA hydrogel. So, it requires various measures to modify the PVA hydrogel. Commonly used methods to change the PVA hydrogel crosslinked water content or conditions, as well as with other materials PVA composite hydrogels, have been used for the composite material hydroxyapatite, ovalbumin, gelatin, fibroin and the like. Through the above method, the mechanical properties of the PVA hydrogel can be improved.

4.4   Contact Surface of Articular Cartilage

In the friction between two solids, the actual contact between the two surfaces occurs on the discrete microprotrusions due to the surface roughness. When the surface microprotrusions are nearby, the forces between the atoms cause the microprotrusions to stick and wear during the mutual friction, and the abrasive particles generated by the wear will further damage the surface. Similarly, for the friction between the cartilage and the artificial joint material, the surface contact state of the cartilage surface with other materials directly affects the frictional properties of the cartilage, so it is necessary to study the surface contact state of the cartilage with other materials.

4.4.1　Laser Scanning Confocal Microscope

Laser scanning confocal microscope (LSCM) is 80 years developed great high-tech products of significance, and is one of the molecular cell biology of the most advanced analytical instruments. It is based on a fluorescence microscope, equipped with a laser scanning device, using a computer for image processing, using ultraviolet light or visible light to excite a fluorescent probe to obtain a fluorescent image of the fine structure inside the cell or tissue, and observing the physiological signal at the subcellular level. And changes in cell morphology provide research assistance in the fields of morphology, molecular cell biology, neuroscience, pharmacology, and heredity. At the same time, laser scanning confocal microscopy can also be applied to other disciplines such as materials science, geology and industrial engineering.

The main components of the LSCM include optical microscope section, laser source, scanning device, detector, computer system (including data acquisition, processing, conversion and application software), image output device and optical device. In a conventional fluorescence microscope, the excitation light from a mercury lamp or a xenon lamp illuminates all the samples in the field of view, and the observer can directly observe with the eyes, or directly use a device such as a CCD to take a fluorescent image. However, the picture obtained by the microscope is susceptible to axial and lateral interference and appears somewhat blurred. For the samples of a certain thickness, on the one hand, since the focal plane of the objective lens in the vertical plane also has fluorescence excited, focal plane fluorescent image plane will have some blurs, which is referred to as axial interference; on the other hand, the samples of the region of these places are also disturbed by fluorescence excited by adjacent regions on the same focal plane, resulting in reduced contrast of the image, which is referred to as lateral interference. The LSCM has some stray light, that is, the dotted line in the schematic diagram, which is not detected by the PMT detector during the imaging process due to the presence of pinholes, thereby improving the imaging effect. A two-dimensional image can be formed by scanning the sample in a point-by-point manner in the x direction and y direction. If the position of the focal plane in the z direction is adjusted and a plurality of two-dimensional images of different z positions are continuously scanned, a 3D image can be formed, and the reconstruction of the specific 3D image requires the support of the corresponding software. In actual operation, the LSCM moves the stage up and down by a micro-stepping motor, and scans the cross-sections of the tissue to obtain images of the respective sections to realize the function of "optical sectioning".

Most LSCMs currently on the market use fluorescence mode, but many non-fluorescent lasers scanning confocal microscopes use confocal bright field technology. Fluorescence laser scanning confocal microscopy has many advantages. It can use special dyes, there is no problem caused by coherent noise, and high-quality three-dimensional images can be obtained. Non-fluorescent reflective laser scanning confocal microscopy bright field lens materials have many applications in science and industry.

4.4.2   Fluorescent Materials and Fluorescence Analysis

After being irradiated with ultraviolet light of certain substances, these substances emit visible light of different colors and intensities. When ultraviolet irradiation is stopped, this light will also disappear soon. This light is called fluorescence. Fluorescence generally includes the visible fluorescence produced by the absorption of ultraviolet light by a substance, and the absorption of a longer wavelength of visible fluorescence after absorption of a shorter wavelength of visible light. The substance absorbs the same photon frequency as its characteristic frequency, and transitions from the original energy level to the different vibrational energy levels and the different rotational energy levels in the first electronically excited state or the second electronically excited state. Most molecules absorb light excited to different vibrational energy after stage and rotational energy levels. The light usually drops sharply to the lowest vibrational level of the first excited electronic state, and it is the process of the same molecule or other molecule collisions that consumes energy equal to the energy between these energy levels. When the lowest vibrational level of the first electronically excited state continues to fall until the different vibrational levels of the ground state, the energy is emitted in the form of light, and the fluorescence is emitted. Using the fluorescence emitted by these substances, qualitative and quantitative analysis of the substance can be performed, which is called fluorescence analysis. There are two kinds of fluorescence of matter. One is spontaneous fluorescence, which is the fluorescence that the tissue emits itself under the illumination of short-wavelength light. The other is the induction of fluorescence, that is, the fluorescence emitted by a certain wavelength of light after the tissue is combined with the fluorescent pigment. It is commonly used for the induction of fluorescence. The fluorescent pigment used is also called fluorescent dye or fluorescent probe, and the fluorescence staining of tissue or cells can be observed on a fluorescence microscope or LSCM equipped with a suitable light source.

4.4.3　Test Method

(1) Sample Preparation

In this test, the human articular cartilage sample was taken first, and then the cartilage sheet was cut with the scalpel parallel cartilage surface. The sample size is approximately 3 mm long, 2 mm wide and 1 mm high. A confocal microscope coverslip having a thickness of 0.17 mm was used as a sample paired with cartilage.

(2) Test Equipment and Steps

The ZEISS LSM 510 META LSCM is a large-scale instrument integrating laser technology, microscope technology, photometric technology, computer and image processing technology, precision mechanical technology, *etc*. In the test, the cartilage was first permeated with physiological saline, and then the glass piece was covered and contacted with the cartilage for observation. The load in the test is the weight of the glass piece itself. There is an amorphous layer on the surface of the cartilage. The amorphous layer contains a large number of glycoproteins, chondroitin, keratan sulfate and proteoglycans, phospholipids, HA and protein aggregates, which have spontaneous fluorescence. In the observation of the confocal microscope, the surface of the cartilage is irradiated with light of a certain wavelength to emit fluorescence, thereby forming a surface fluorescence image.

4.4.4　Test Results

The result is a picture of contact between the cartilage surface and glass body (see Figure 4-5 and Figure 4-6 before contents). As can be seen from the result, the surface of the articular cartilage is undulating. After the light is irradiated, the fluorescence is emitted, and the surface fluorescence picture is obtained, the fluorescence distribution is not uniform. A slice of the contact area between the cartilage and the glass was obtained by observing the z direction slice. Place C has a continuous fluorescence distribution on the whole slice surface, and discontinuities appear at A and B. The discontinuous part is that the concave portion of the cartilage surface is not in contact with the glass. It can be seen that in the contact surface of cartilage and glass, part of the cartilage and glass are not in effective contact. The glass has a smooth and flat surface, and the surface of the cartilage has a certain height and undulation. The presence of the uncontacted area of cartilage and glass may be related to the fluctuation of the surface of the cartilage.

4.5   Analysis of the Influence of Articular Cartilage Surface Contact on Friction Performance

In the study of Kobayashi & Oka (2003), the contact state of rabbit articular cartilage with 0.15 mm thick glass surface was observed by laser confocal microscopy. The load applied in the test was 12 N, which was equivalent to the physiological load of the rabbit in daily exercise. After loading the normal cartilage surface, the contact area is divided into two areas: one is the contact area, the cartilage surface is in direct contact with the glass piece, and the other is the liquid pool area with a liquid film between them. Under saline lubrication, the liquid film area surrounds the contact area, and the cartilage surface depression is rarely found. The intermediate zone between the two zones has a transition zone. Kobayashi and others believe that the transition zone is under load. This area is composed of macromolecules such as protein and HA. Macromolecules such as protein and HA have polarities. Under high pressure, they form liquid crystal molecules, which support physiological load. At the same time, it can act as a boundary lubricant to reduce the adhesion of the friction interface.

In the test of this subject, the human articular cartilage and the glass were tested. There was no external physiological load in the test. The weight of the glass sample was pressed against the cartilage surface, and the load was much smaller than the load in the Kobayashi study. It is shown by LSCM in the z direction that there is a glass region in the direct contact area, which can not be found in the middle of the transition zone. It is shown that cartilage slices contacting with the glass region can be seen, and the contact surface is continuous in some regions, such as Region C. The region will have some disconnecting phenomena, such as A and B areas. The results showed that it is similar for the glass in contact with the cartilage solid interface asperity contacting during rubbing, and the joint smooth surface area of cartilage which is in contact with the glass is discontinuous. Many wide areas with several micrometers are not in contact with each other. This may be related to the natural depressions on the cartilage surface, which form a pool of liquid that stores a large amount of lubricating fluid. It is beneficial to provide a lubricating fluid to reduce friction when the cartilage is under load.

4. 6 Summary

This chapter firstly compares the biomechanical properties of human articular cartilage, bovine articular cartilage and PVA hydrogel artificial cartilage. Compressive stress-strain, stress relaxation, and creep tests were carried out to obtain the stress-strain relationship of human articular cartilage, bovine articular cartilage and PVA hydrogel artificial cartilage. It was found that the stress state of the same PVA hydrogel bovine articular cartilage strain is greater than other materials. The material of minimum strain values is human articular cartilage. The compressive modulus of the articular cartilage was 3.6492 ± 0.6199 MPa, and the compressive modulus of PVA hydrogel was 1.5951 ± 0.1469 MPa. The compression modulus of bovine articular cartilage was 2.7645 ± 0.3667 MPa. In the creep test, the strain of human cartilage changed more value than that of the PVA hydrogel, and the stress of the human cartilage in the stress relaxation test also changed from the initial value to higher value. The change of bovine cartilage was between human cartilage and PVA hydrogel.

The composition and internal structure of artificial cartilage and natural cartilage lead to their different mechanical properties. In order to make artificial cartilage closer to natural cartilage, it is necessary to improve the mechanical properties of PVA hydrogel, which requires various measures for PVA water. The gel is modified. It is commonly used method to change the PVA hydrogel crosslinked water content or conditions, as well as other materials, to produce PVA composite hydrogels. It is important to improve the structure of the PVA hydrogel because internal void distribution is more regular.

The surface contact state of the cartilage and the artificial joint material directly affects the friction between them. In this chapter, the glass of the same hard material as the artificial joint material is used instead, and the surface contact state of the cartilage and the glass is observed. It can be found from the experiment that the contact between the cartilage surface and the glass is irregular and is affected by the natural high and low fluctuations of the cartilage surface. The z direction scan of the LSCM revealed a direct contact zone and a liquid pool zone of the cartilage-glass contact area. The contact between the cartilage and the glass is similar to the contact of the two solid interfaces in the micro convex contact during the friction process. The contact area between the articular cartilage and the smooth surface of the glass is discontinuous, and many of the regions with a width of several tens of micrometers are not in contact with each other, which may be related to the natural depressions on the cartilage surface. The liquid pool area formed by these recessed areas stores a large amount of lubricating liquid, which provides a lubricating fluid to reduce friction when the cartilage is under load.

Chapter 5
Friction Behavior of Natural and Artificial Cartilage

5.1   Introduction

In the study of biotribology area, the researchers do research on cartilage, which is mainly focused on the friction between natural cartilage and natural cartilage, as well as the friction between artificial joint materials, such as the friction between UHMWPE and cobalt-chromium molybdenum alloy. The other is the modification of artificial joint materials. After several decades of development, it has been difficult for the frictional properties between artificial joint materials to further increase, so researchers begin to design artificial joints from the perspective of natural joints, including the "cushion-supported artificial joints" proposed by Professor Dowson of the United Kingdom.

An important feature of the cushion-supported artificial joint is that the artificial joint material no longer adheres to the use of cemented carbide or polymer materials, such as cobalt-chromium molybdenum, ceramics and titanium alloys. A lot of new materials are used, which are selected from the perspective of bionic bionics. For the bionics of cartilage, it mainly includes three important aspects: structural bionics, material bionics and functional bionics. The structure bionics mainly manifests as the porous permeability and composite gradient structure of the material; the material bionic performance is self-lubricating, low elastic modulus and biological connection. The functional bionic performance is able to withstand and transfer load, good wear resistance and self-lubrication performance. In response to these bionic requirements, Professor Peppas first proposed the use of PVA as a material for artificial joints in 1977. The processing of PVA to obtain polyethylene hydrogel has been greatly improved as a new generation of artificial joint materials. There is a great development in using conventional artificial joint cartilage materials. New artificial joint hydrogel material such as polyethylene has been used to conduct the reciprocating rotational friction test. The research between cartilage and artificial joint material has provided the basis for further improvement of artificial cartilage material.

5.2   Development of Dual-Purpose Friction Testing Machine

5.2.1   Common Reciprocating Friction Testing Machine

Common sliding tests for sliding contact have three main types of contact, namely point contact (ball to disk or plane), line contact (cylinder to disk or plane) and curved surface contact (planar and plane). Commonly used friction testing machines mainly include a four-ball machine, a ring block testing machine, a double-plate contact fatigue testing machine, a reciprocating friction and pin-type friction testing machine, *etc.*, which are mostly designed for a certain type of friction test. Due to the variety of frictional motions, it is necessary to better design the friction tester to accommodate a wide range of test requirements.

Researchers from different countries have developed a number of small reciprocating friction rub testers, which have their own characteristics. The friction test device used by Yu Zhenglin can measure the friction characteristics of micron-scale samples and require two sets of laser light sources, which requires high technical conditions and high cost. Li Zhiheng designed a friction rub test micro-test device. The testing machine with a sample loading force of the lever, and with the front end of the arm to measure and square this formula is directly connected to the measured sample arm. The protection of the force arm and the deformation of the force arm also have an effect on the friction measurement. Forsey, Fisher, Thompson, Stone, Bell & Ingham (2006) used HA and phospholipids as lubricants to affect the cartilage of damaged human cartilage. A reciprocating linear friction test device was used in the test. The test configuration can effectively measure the friction force of the reciprocating movement.

5.2.2   Test Requirements

In this topic, we mainly study the friction and wear of natural and artificial joint materials. The movement of the natural knee and hip joints is a combination of rolling and sliding. Therefore, the reciprocating friction method can be used to partially simulate the motion of the natural joint to test the performance of the joint material. For natural cartilage in living organisms, due to the need to perform certain physiological functions in the organism, it has the following characteristics.

First, the shape is irregular. The articular cartilage of the mammal bears the bearing and lubrication function of the joint and covers the surface of the joint surface. Therefore, the articular cartilage itself is also a curved surface. For the friction test, the sample with a large shape and a large length cannot be obtained when the sample is taken. The traditional friction test is carried out, and the same problem exists for other natural biological materials. In view of the above, there is a need for a testing machine that can be used for friction testing of small samples.

Second, for biomaterials, the weight they bear within their functional range is lightly loaded, and the current testing machines are mainly heavy loads.

Third, biomaterials need to be supported by simulations of the physiological environment, which requires the provision of appropriate devices to maintain the *in vivo* environment required by the biomaterial.

One of the original testing machines in this research uses the rotation of the cam to drive the sample back and forth. The testing machine can only perform the relevant wear test, and there is no reagent tank for the lubricating fluid. It is now modified for the requirements of this study.

The modified testing machine can measure the frictional force in both directions of reciprocating motion and maintain the lubrication environment required by biological materials. A sample slot is mounted on the single-coordinate reciprocating platform driven by the cam in the testing machine, and the lower sample is installed on the bottom of the sample slot. The sample slot is processed by medical stainless steel material, and the physiological liquid is placed in the groove to immerse the biological material sample. A heating device is installed to maintain a constant temperature during the test. The testing machine realizes a dual-purpose machine, one is to perform a reciprocating linear motion friction test, and the other is to perform a reciprocating rotational friction test of the sample. Reciprocating linear motion is produced by using a cam implemented. The reciprocating rotational has used the rack and pinion structure of the tester to convert reciprocating motion into rotation. Two test methods are shown in the result. Tester physical map and real-time measurement map are also given (see Figure 5-1).

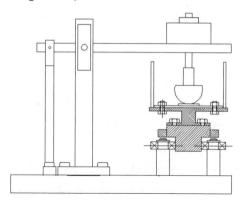

Figure 5-1   Schematic Illustrations of Two Test Methods

(1) Mechanical Structure

In the reciprocating test, the upper sample is directly mounted on the lower end of the vertical rod, the lower sample is mounted on the bottom of the sample groove during the reciprocating linear motion test, and the lower sample is mounted on the top of the reciprocating shaft during the reciprocating rotational motion. The lubricating fluid is immersed in the tank to immerse the sample. A rack-mounted sample reciprocating direction of the rack with the upper gear tooth bar driven with reciprocating motion of the reciprocating gear rotates, and the reciprocating rotary motion is transmitted to the gear to the next sample by a gear shaft mounted on the shaft. The horizontal rod and the reciprocating platform are placed at 90 degrees, the vertical rod is installed at the front end of the horizontal rod, the lower end of the vertical rod is mounted with a sample, and the upper end of the vertical rod is mounted with a weight as a load. The horizontal rod is supported at the rear by a support rod that is perpendicular to the tabletop, and the horizontal rod is horizontally and vertically movable around the support rod.

The connecting block is a square hollow lightweight block with a single screw installed at one end. The screw is rotated until the screw head is lightly pressed against the end of the horizontal rod, and then the screw is used to fix the screw position. The other end of the connecting block is connected to the force sensor by a screw, and the other end of the force sensor is connected to the mounting plate of the fixed force sensor. The rear end of the horizontal rod projects into the connecting block, and the force sensor is generated by the connecting block.

(2) Force Measurement Method

The commonly used force measurement methods in the test are as follows: ① The measured force can be directly measured by the known gravity or electromagnetic force to balance the measured force; ② Measuring a force acting on the measured force, the acceleration of the known mass object is used to indirectly measure the measured force; ③ The measured force is measured by measuring the fluid pressure generated by the measured force; ④ The vibrating string is tensioned by the measured force, the natural frequency of the string is changed with the magnitude of the measured force, and the measured force is measured by measuring the change of the frequency; ⑤ The measured force is measured by measuring the deformation or strain of an elastic element under the force of the measured force. The first four measurement methods are mainly used for the measurement of static force or slowly varying force, and the fifth can be used for static force or measurement of dynamic force below several kilohertz. In this subject, the reciprocating tester is designed for the friction and wear of natural and artificial cartilage materials. The reciprocating speed is in accordance with the moving speed of the human body in daily life. The frictional force with the reciprocating motion always changes in two directions, mainly within ten hertz, tests carried out using a measuring force fifth embodiment.

The mechanical measurement system of this testing machine is mainly composed of the Z6 force sensor of Germany HBM, the signal amplification module AD101B and the data processing and communication module AED9101B. The measurement system is connected to the host computer through the serial port. The axial tension (pressure) of the sensor is allowed to be less than 10 kg. The lateral force is allowed to be less than 10 kg, and the dynamic force is less than 5 kg, which can meet the test requirements. In the reciprocating friction test, the friction between the samples is amplified by the lever, and the force of the horizontal rod is detected by the force sensor placed vertically to obtain the frictional force. During the test, the signal measured by the force sensor is subjected to signal amplification and data processing, the change of the measured force is displayed on the screen in real-time through communication with the host computer, and the result can be stored in real-time.

(3) Test Method

When the friction test was conducted by rotational movement, the surface of the specimen mounted at the counterpart material. The platform was conducted with reciprocated motion. The sample was racked from the bottom with reciprocally-rotated testing. The reciprocating gear transformed through the gear shaft. The rotary motion is transmitted to the sample under reciprocating rotational motion mounted on the shaft. During the friction process, the friction force of the upper sample is compressed or stretched by the lever amplification of the horizontal rod, and the force of the connecting block is transmitted to the force sensor through the force sensor fixing screw and the positioning screw to generate a signal.

When the reciprocating linear motion friction test is carried out, the sample is directly installed at the bottom of the sample tank under the reciprocating linear motion, and the reciprocating platform drives the sample to reciprocate linearly under the reciprocating linear motion in the sample groove, and the friction of the upper sample during the friction process after leverage force amplification lever for compression or tension generated on the connecting block. The force transmitted to the connection block of the force sensor signals being generated by the force sensor fixing screw.

5.3   Reciprocating Linear Motion Friction Test

5.3.1   Test Method

In order to study the friction characteristics of cartilage and common cartilage materials under load, speed and lubrication changes, the reciprocating linear motion friction test and the reciprocating rotary motion friction test were carried out using the established dual-purpose friction tester. The reciprocating linear motion friction test uses two pairs of cartilage and stainless steel, and cartilage and PVA hydrogel artificial cartilage.

(1) Sample Preparation

Using the same sample processing method, the obtained samples were bovine articular cartilage and PVA hydrogel. Bovine articular cartilage specimens were a diameter of 9 mm pin sample, the PVA hydrogel was obtained by a chemical crosslinking method, and 15% the PVA was dissolved in 80% of DMSO solution obtained by freeze-thawing. The stainless steel is 317 L medical stainless steel with a surface roughness of $Ra = 0.05$.

(2) Test Equipment

The ESEM pair was used in the test. ESEM is a product of FEI Company of the

United States, model number XL30. ESEM and AFM were used in the observation of abrasive grains. The AFM used the Nanoscope-III AFM of American DI Company of Shanghai Jiaotong University. In the energy spectrum analysis, the Genesis type spectrometer with ESEM was used for correlation analysis. Particle size analysis of the abrasive particles was also carried out using LS13320 laser particle size analyzer (Beckman Coulter Inc.).

(3)Test Procedure

The reciprocating linear motion friction test stroke was 14 mm, and an orthogonal test of a total of eight test conditions was performed. Three test conditions were performed for each test condition, the frictional force at 3 minutes was measured, and the friction coefficient was calculated by calculation. After the factor test, a test combination was selected for the long-term friction test of 120 minutes to observe the change of the friction coefficient and the change of the surface of the sample. In this test, the selected load is 22 N, the speed is 10 mm/s, the long-term lubrication friction test mode is a combination of these couples saline or HA, and the use of long-term friction test ESEM surface topography with physiological saline lubrication is observed. The abrasive particles after long-term friction between cartilage and stainless steel were analyzed. The temperature was kept at room temperature during the test. The three factors of load, speed and lubrication are shown in Table 5-1.

Table 5-1　Test Parameters

Factor	Level 1	Level 2
Load (N)	10	22
Speed (mm/s)	10	20
Lubricating	Ringer solution	HA (2.5 g/L)

The joint load range of the human body in daily life is about 0–5 MPa, wherein the contact stress of the hip joint under normal conditions is about 1.4–2.9 MPa, and the maximum contact stress can reach 9.57 MPa in extreme cases. When a person walks normally, the average speed of movement between the acetabulum and the ball head in the hip joint is 1–2 rad/s, and the linear velocity is 0–0.1 m/s. It is a better friction and wear mechanisms of articular cartilage to facilitate comparison between different materials, selected in this test contained in the normal daily life test charge. The test used is a form of cartilage pin reciprocating friction. The pin sample has a diameter of 9 mm and a cross-sectional area of about 63.6 mm^2. It can be seen from the calculation that when the applied load is 10 N, the contact stress of the friction pair is about 0.16 MPa , and the contact stress at the load of 22 N is 0.35 MPa. Since the joint speed of the human body is low at most times, the speed is selected to be 10 mm/s and 20 mm/s in the test, and the cartilage friction is in the boundary lubrication and mixed lubrication state in this speed range (Brand, 2005; Forster & Fisher, 1999).

OA is a chronic degenerative joint disease that is a group of diseases with different causes but similar biological, morphological and clinical manifestations. The disease affects the articular cartilage and lesions and injuries occur throughout the joint. Clinical manifestations are slow joint swelling, stiffness and limited mobility, as well as secondary synovitis. The main component of the synovial fluid and cartilage matrix is HA. Studies have shown that the concentration of HA in the joint cavity of OA is significantly lower than that of healthy people. Peyron & Balazs (1974) first proposed the injection of exogenous HA to treat OA, and the American College of Rheumatology further advocated the use of HA as a means of treating OA (Altman, Hochberg, Moskowitz & Schnitzer, 2000). In this test, HA was used as a comparative lubricant with physiological saline, and the concentration of the solution was in the concentration range of HA in human joint fluid. The HA used in the test was produced by Chia Tai Group with a molecular weight of 2×10^6 Da.

5.3.2   Friction Properties of Cartilage and Stainless Steel

(1) Effects of Load, Speed and Lubrication

The result shows the change in the friction coefficient between cartilage and stainless steel under different loading conditions (see Figure 5-2). It can be seen that the friction coefficient between cartilage and stainless steel decreases with increasing load under the same speed and lubrication conditions. When the test is in saline lubrication with a speed of 10 mm/s, if the load from 10 N increased to 22 N, the coefficient of friction between the cartilage and the stainless steel decreased from 0.147 down to 0.117. At the same time, it can be seen that the friction coefficient between the cartilage and the stainless steel decreases more with the increase of the load at a lower speed. The result shows the change in the friction coefficient between cartilage and stainless steel at different speeds. It can be seen that under the same lubrication and pressure, the higher the speed, the smaller the friction coefficient of cartilage and stainless steel. Under the conditions of load 10 N and saline as lubrication, the friction coefficient obtained in the test was reduced from 0.148 to 0.105. It also shows the effect of lubrication on the coefficient of friction between cartilage and stainless steel. It can be seen that the HA solution can effectively reduce the friction between the cartilage and the stainless steel. Under the load of 10 N and the reciprocating speed of 10 mm/s, the friction coefficient of cartilage and stainless steel under the lubrication of physiological saline is 0.148, and the friction coefficient is reduced to 0.132 under the lubrication of HA solution. In the previous study, a reciprocating friction test was carried out using a bovine cartilage pin and a bovine cartilage piece as a matching pair. It was found that the friction coefficient between cartilage and cartilage gradually decreased as the load increased from 0.2 MPa to 0.4 MPa. In the test of this subject, when the load is increased between the bovine cartilage and the stainless steel, the friction coefficient becomes small.

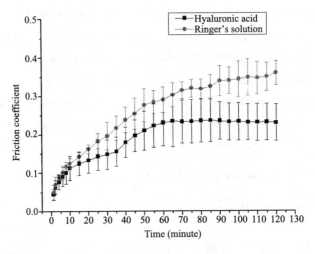

Figure 5-2   The Change of Friction Coefficient

(2) Long-Term Friction Test

The result shows the results between cartilage and stainless steel under 22 N load in 120 minutes. It can be seen that the friction coefficient between the cartilage and the stainless steel is constantly changing in the two lubrication states as the test time progresses. Two kinds of lubrication have different effects on the friction coefficient. So the trends can be seen from the result, the coefficient of friction of cartilage and stainless steel in saline always increased with the same lubrication, and the friction coefficient at the start is 0.05 or less, and the front 50 minutes of the friction coefficient has more rapid rise. In the HA lubrication, the friction coefficient changes in cartilage and smoother stainless steel, which results in no difference in the coefficient of friction at the start.

5.3.3   Wear Observation of Cartilage and Stainless Steel

(1) Surface Morphology Observation

The result shows an ESEM image of the surface of the bovine cartilage test, which is the surface of the bovine cartilage that has worn out (see Figure 5-3). It can be seen that after a long-term friction test a large amount of wear particles appears on the surface of the cartilage, the surface of the cartilage has an uneven surface, and the surface has obvious scratches.

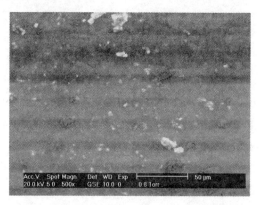

Figure 5-3   ESEM Image of Bovine Cartilage after Test

(2) Wear Particle Observation

After the cartilage and the stainless steel were continuously rubbed for 120 minutes, the abrasive grains obtained after the test were observed. The results are views of abrasive particles using AFM and ESEM (see Figure 5-4), respectively. As can be seen from the AFM chart, the shape of the abrasive grains is relatively regular, and the abrasive grains are similar in shape to a spherical shape. In the result, the larger diameter abrasive grains produced by the test were observed by ESEM, and it was found that the surface of the abrasive grains was rough and had minute protrusions. The result is a graph showing the size distribution of the abrasive grains obtained by using the LS13320 laser particle size analyzer. It can be seen that the particle size distribution range of the abrasive grains is narrow, the size of the abrasive grains is mainly concentrated between 0 and 4, and the number of small-sized abrasive grains is large.

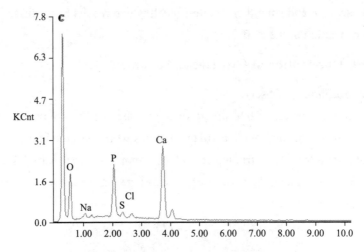

Figure 5-4　EDX Analysis of Wear Particles

(3) Abrasive Element Analysis

The result shows the results of an energy spectrum analysis of the surface of the bovine cartilage after abrasion. The particles contain 4.22% by weight of phosphorus and 9.3% by weight of calcium, the elemental composition of the surface of the unworn bovine cartilage has been measured to contain 0.23% by weight of phosphorus and 0.52% by weight of calcium, and the surface of the cartilage is observed to be worn. It can be seen that there are higher phosphorus particles and the content of calcium, and the cartilage surface is unworn 10 times, indicating that serious damage to the cartilage surface.

5.3.4　Cartilage and PVA Hydrogel Friction Properties

(1) Effects of Load, Speed and Lubrication

The result is a schematic diagram of the effect of the friction coefficient on the load during the reciprocating friction of cartilage and PVA hydrogel (see Figure 5-5). It can be seen that the greater the load during the friction process, the greater the coefficient of friction between the cartilage and the PVA hydrogel. When the load between the cartilage and the PVA hydrogel is 10 N and is lubricated with physiological saline, and the reciprocating speed is 10 mm/s, the friction coefficient is 0.12. At the same reciprocating speed, the friction coefficient is reduced to 0.084 when the load becomes 22 N. The result shows the coefficient of friction changed between the cartilage and PVA hydrogel by the impact of the moving speed. It can be seen that under the same lubrication and load conditions, when the reciprocating speed of the cartilage pin increases, the friction coefficient between the cartilage and the PVA hydrogel becomes larger. When the load is 10 N, saline lubricated between the cartilage and the PVA hydrogel increases from 0.12 to 0.147. The result shows the effect of lubrication on the friction coefficient between the cartilage and the PVA hydrogel. It can be seen that HA can effectively reduce the friction between cartilage and PVA hydrogel. When the load is 10 N, the speed is 10 mm/s, and the lubrication condition is changed into the HA, the friction coefficient decreases from 0.12 down to 0.114.

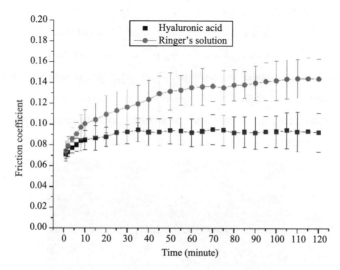

Figure 5-5   The Change of Friction Coefficient

(2) Long-Term Friction Test

The result shows the results of a 120-minute friction test of cartilage and PVA hydrogel. It can be seen that under the saline lubrication, the friction coefficient between the cartilage and the PVA hydrogel is always increasing, and the rising trend of the friction coefficient is always changing. The first 15 minutes has the fastest increase, at the rest of the time the coefficient of friction increases slowly, and the coefficient of friction after 90 minutes fluctuates between 0.14 and 0.15. When the cartilage and the PVA hydrogel were moved under the lubrication of HA, the friction coefficient increased at the beginning. But after 20 minutes, it began to stabilize at around 0.092. It can be seen from the above comparison that HA can effectively reduce the friction between cartilage and PVA hydrogel, and can help the friction pair to enter a stable state with a relatively low friction coefficient.

5.3.5 Observation of Cartilage and PVA Hydrogel Wear

The result is an ESEM image of the surface after the bovine cartilage test (see Figure 5-6). It can be seen that there are no obvious pits on the surface of bovine cartilage, the surface has some undulations, and a small number of wear particles appear, and there is material accumulation on the surface of the cartilage. It can be induced that the amorphous layer on the surface of the cartilage is gathered in the friction tests. The results are the ESEM images of the surface after the PVA hydrogel test. It has been found from the drawing, the PVA porous structure surface of the hydrogel in its original state has disappeared, and the surface shows many serious scratches with cutting traces. Due to the lower modulus and tear resistance, the surface of the PVA hydrogel is tractable. PVA original surface of the hydrogel has been peeled, and because the inside of the porous layer structure is exposed, the porous layer-like structure is affected by surface contact friction test stress, which also induces material failure. It can be seen that a mesh-like surface is created.

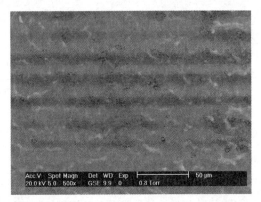

Figure 5-6   ESEM Images of PVA Hydrogel After Test

The result shows an ESEM image of surface adhesion after bovine cartilage testing (see Figure 5-7). As can be seen from the result, a large amount of adherent adheres to the surface of the bovine cartilage. The results are partially enlarged views. The cartilage has adhered near the edge of the area, and adhesive attachment was irregular in shape, which is the sheet-like presentation layer. The result is an enlarged view of the adherent. The structure of the adherent can be seen from the result. There are a large number of holes in the adherent, and it has a translucent appearance. Through the surface the lower cartilage layer can be seen. Fragmentation occurs at the same time. The result shows the results of the elemental analysis of the surface of the adherend by an energy spectrometer. Compared with the surface elemental composition of natural cartilage, the elemental composition in the adherend is consistent with the cartilage surface, and the element content is not much different. When the elemental composition of the material and the porous structure of the surface are examined, the material appears as a part of the surface, which may be caused by the wear of the PVA hydrogel. PVA hydrogel has the macromolecular chain of the hydrogel that occurs on sliding wear hydrogel nature. Thereby the test changed the surface of the hydrogel, and the gel sheet material the surface of the water transfer moved surface of a coupling member, which causes adhesive wear.

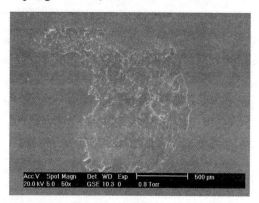

Figure 5-7   ESEM Image of Surface Adhesion of Bovine Cartilage

5.4   Analysis of Friction and Wear Mechanism of Reciprocating Linear Motion

5.4.1   Cartilage and Stainless Steel

(1) Impact of the Load

In the reciprocating friction test between cartilage and stainless steel, the friction coefficient decreases as the load increases. Under low load, the load borne by the cartilage two-phase structure, most of the load is sustained by the liquid phase, which is advantageous in maintaining low friction in cartilage. When the load is increased, the liquid cartilage bears most of the load again. In the model calculation (Katta, Pawaskar, Jin, Ingham & Fisher, 2007), it has been found that when the contact stress of the cartilage surface does not exceed 0.4 MPa, the load on the cartilage increases. The load on the liquid phase in the cartilage at the same time keeps increasing but mainly occurring in the total load. The percentage has remained the same, and it can be said that the proportion of the load that the solid phase is subjected to remains unchanged. For the case in this test, the solid phase in the cartilage can also maintain a fixed proportion of load during the load increase, which will result in a constant coefficient of friction. However, with the increase in the load test, the coefficient of friction between the stainless steel decreases. The friction coefficient can be seen not only in the ratio of the carrier about the solid phase, possibly directly related to the surface condition of the cartilage.

The surface of cartilage and stainless steel has a certain roughness. The average roughness of bovine cartilage is $Ra = 1.37$, and the surface roughness of stainless steel is $Ra = 0.05$. The roughness of the two is quite different. The size of the peaks and valleys of the surface of bovine cartilage is larger than that of the stainless steel surface. The elastic modulus of stainless steel is 206 GPa, which is much larger than the elastic modulus of cartilage. The different hardness of the two materials will affect the friction characteristics between them. During the friction process, the cartilage interacts with the micro convex peaks and valleys on the surface of the stainless steel. The micro convex peaks on the surface of the cartilage are not only high in height but also low in hardness. The peaks of the cartilage surface will be deformed and flattened during the contact between the two surfaces. The cut material will further fill the valley of the surface, and the deformation or flattening of the peak will make the surface of the cartilage smoother, resulting in lower roughness. When the load increases, the peak of the cartilage surface will bear a greater load, which will aggravate the deformation and flattening of the peak. The cartilage surface will be smoother than the smaller load, so the friction coefficient will be reduced.

(2) The Effect of Speed and Lubrication

The surface contact between cartilage and stainless steel at different speeds is similar, and the contact area between the two surfaces mainly contains micro convex peaks and valleys. The contact state of the two surfaces is mainly determined by the characteristics of the material of the cartilage surface, wherein the deformation and flattening of the micro convex peak directly affect the change in the surface roughness of the cartilage. Under the same amount of load, the deformation speed of the micro convex peak on the cartilage surface is the same under different loading speeds. The tensile stress of the micro convex body per unit time in the reciprocating direction will increase, which will lead to micro convex at high speed. The increase in peak flattening damage, and the cartilage surface will be smoother and smoother when the speed is high, and the resistance to the movement will be reduced, so the friction coefficient will be reduced.

HA is widely present in animal and human tissues and the extracellular matrix body. The synovial fluid viscoelasticity is associated with HA. HA itself is not subjected to load, and it reorganizes the water by its internal structure to achieve load-bearing and improved lubrication. HA forms a network structure in space, and water molecules are combined with HA molecules through polar bonds and hydrogen bonds in the network. So, the water is fixed inside, and the HA solution is used as lubrication in the reciprocating friction test. The agent is beneficial for maintaining moisture between the samples and is beneficial for reducing friction.

(3) Wear

A large amount of wear particles can be observed from the ESEM photograph of the cartilage surface after the test, the surface of the cartilage has an uneven surface, and the surface has obvious scratches. In the test results, it is shown that cartilage and stainless steel mainly have abrasive wear. The surface fatigue and wear are under sliding wear conditions. In the friction pair composed of cartilage and stainless steel, the microprotrusions on the surface of the cartilage are in contact with the stainless steel surface at various angles under the external load. When the microprotrusion forms a favorable angle of attack with the surface of the stainless steel, the shear force is applied, and micro-cutting action occurs, which is forming debris; the surface of the negative angle of attack is formed, and the wear occurs when the cartilage surface forms a large deformation. Under the action of the furrow's asperity, the surface material of the cartilage is easily worn away. When the wear is occurring, the surface of the cartilage deforms, which is due to the continuous action of cyclic stress. When the deformation of the worn surface reaches a certain level, the deformed layer may generate cracks. After the crack is formed, under the action of the frictional stress, the crack expands, which is eventually leading to the peeling of the cartilage surface material.

5.4.2   Cartilage and PVA Hydrogel

(1) Impact of Load

In the reciprocating friction test between cartilage and PVA hydrogel, the friction coefficient decreases as the load increases. When the load is increased, the contact stress of the cartilage pin and the PVA hydrogel becomes large, and the deformation of the PVA hydrogel becomes large. The mode of motion in this test is reciprocating motion. The contact surface of the PVA hydrogel with the cartilage pin is fixed, and the contact surface on the PVA hydrogel is not always loaded. When the surface of the PVA hydrogel contacts the cartilage pin, it will deform, and part of the liquid phase absorbed inside will go out from the surface hole. The exuded liquid phase is beneficial to improve the lubrication of the friction pair; when the surface of the PVA hydrogel is not in contact, the PVA hydrogel recovers under the action of elastic force. The part of the liquid phase is absorbed into the body during the recovery process. When the load becomes larger, the deformation of the surface of the PVA hydrogel in contact with the cartilage pin is increased, and the amount of the liquid phase oozing out from the pores of the PVA hydrogel surface is also increased, which is more advantageous for the lubrication of the friction pair. Therefore, the friction coefficient is further reduced compared to the loaded hour.

(2) The Effect of Speed and Lubrication

In the reciprocating friction test between cartilage and PVA hydrogel, the friction coefficient increases as the sliding speed increases. The reasons are mainly manifested in two aspects. Firstly, the change of sliding speed will cause the surface of the friction pair to change. With the increase of speed, the surface of PVA hydrogel is more prone to deformation and flow, and the ability of the material to resist shear deformation decreases. This will accelerate and aggravate the wear of the PVA hydrogel. Secondly, the sliding speed has a large effect on the two-phase performance of the PVA hydrogel. When the slide is at low moving speed, the PVA hydrogel with no recovery time becomes a long cartilage pin, and a large amount of distortion recovery phase is re-absorbed, which is conducive to reduce friction. When the sliding speed increases, the recovery time of the PVA hydrogel decreases. The degree of deformation recovery and the amount of liquid re-absorption are reduced, which are not conducive to reducing friction, so the friction coefficient is higher than the value when the sliding speed is low. In the reciprocating friction test of cartilage and PVA hydrogel, HA solution as a lubricant can effectively reduce the friction coefficient of the friction pair.

(3) Wear

It can be seen from the test results that cartilage and PVA hydrogel mainly have two kinds of wear modes: adhesive wear and surface fatigue wear. These phenomena occur under reciprocating friction conditions. It is known from the mechanical tests that have been carried out that the elastic modulus of cartilage is larger than that of PVA hydrogel. When the test case in the experiment is subjected to the same load, the ability of PVA hydrogel to resist the deformation of the surface of the hydrogel is weak, and the cartilage surface is less than the deformation of PVA modified hydrogel when contacted asperity occurs. PVA hydrogel surface peaks are stripped under shear and the fragments are separated. Under the effect of compressive stress, the isolated PVA hydrogel debris progressively decreases the cartilage surface of the transfer phase, which increases the roughness of the contact surface of the sticking.

When the wear is in processing, under the action of cyclic stress, the PVA hydrogel matrix is in front of the microprotrusion in a compressed state, the compressive stress does not cause the formation and expansion of cracks and scratches, and the rear matrix is in a tensile stress state. The surface is covered with holes, which will result in tensile stresses in the PVA hydrogel weakness in the hole formed into the crack, and the crack is extended further, and final tearing of the surface pores fatigue wear occurs.

5.5   Reciprocating Rotary Motion Friction Test

5.5.1   Test Method

(1) Sample Preparation and Test Equipment

In the experiments, the friction characteristic of cartilage in joints and artificial ceramic material is examined, and the dual-friction reciprocating rotational motion rub testing machine is used for testing. The hip ceramic ball head (BIOLOX® forte, Ceram Tec AG., Germany) was used in the test. The material was aluminum oxide with a roughness of 0.02 micron and a diameter of 28 mm. Specimens include some pins of bovine articular with 9 mm diameter.

(2) Test Procedure

In the reciprocating rotational motion of the testing machine, the reciprocating platform speed is 10 mm/s, which is equal to the rotational speed of the ball 0.3125 rad/s, and the ball in terms of rotation circumference is 12.25 mm. The three factors which are load, speed and lubrication are used in the test, which is the same as those in the reciprocating linear motion. According to the Hertz contact formula, when the applied load is 10 N, the contact stress of the friction pair is about 0.64 MPa , and the contact stress is equal to 0.81 MPa when the load is 22 N.

A total of 8 test conditions were subjected to the orthogonal test, each test condition was made in 3 groups, the frictional force at 3 minutes was measured, and the friction coefficient was calculated by calculation. Factors then were used in the tests of 120 minutes, and the friction coefficient of variation was observed. When the test load is 22 N and the speed is 10 mm/s, the long-term friction tests include lubrication of a combination of physiological saline or HA. Then ESEM is used to examine the surface morphology while sub-lubrication saline was observed, and elemental analysis of the worn particles.

5.5.2　Cartilage and Ceramic Ball Head Friction Properties

(1) Effects of Load, Speed and Lubrication

The change of friction coefficient between the cartilage and the ceramic ball head under different loads is shown (see Figure 5-8). It can be seen that under the same speed and lubrication conditions, the friction coefficient between the cartilage and the ceramic ball head decreases as the load increases. When samples were in saline lubrication with a speed 10 mm/s, as the load increased from 10 N to 22 N, the coefficient of friction between the cartilage and the ceramic ball head decreased from 0.068 down to 0.049. The change of friction properties between the cartilage and the ceramic ball head affected by the movement speed is shown. It can be seen that under the same load and lubrication conditions, the friction coefficient between the cartilage

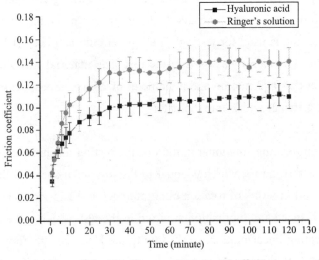

Figure 5-8　The Change of Friction Coefficient

and the ceramic ball head increases as the moving speed increases at the same time. When the load is 10 N and the speed is increased from 10 mm/s to 20 mm/s, the friction coefficient of the friction pair increases from 0.068 to 0.093 under the lubrication of physiological saline. The result shows the effect of lubrication on the frictional properties between the cartilage and the ceramic ball head. As can be seen from the results, the friction coefficient of the friction pair using HA as a lubricant is lower than that obtained by physiological saline lubrication under the same test conditions.

(2) Long-Term Friction Test

The result shows the change in the coefficient of friction between the cartilage and ceramic ball head during a 120-minute reciprocating frictional motion. As can be seen from the result, the cartilage and ceramic ball head experienced a process in which the friction coefficient first rises rapidly and then rises slowly under both lubrication conditions, in which the friction coefficient rises faster in the first 30 minutes. The friction coefficient of the friction pair lubricated with HA in 120 minutes is always smaller than that of the friction pair which is lubricated with physiological saline.

5.5.3　Wear Observation of Cartilage and Ceramic Ball Head

The result is an ESEM observation of the surface of the bovine cartilage in tests (see Figure 5-9). It can be seen that the surface of the cartilage has revealed an uneven structure, many large pieces of wear particles appear on the surface of the samples, and some surface areas of the cartilage appear to be damaged.

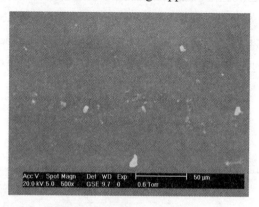

Figure 5-9　ESEM Image of Bovine Cartilage After the Test

The result shows of an energy spectrum analysis of the surface of the bovine cartilage after abrasion (see Figure 5-10). The results showed that the particles contained 3.96% by weight of phosphorus and 8.05% by weight of calcium, both of which far exceeded the elements of the untreated bovine cartilage surface. This shows that during rubbing, the cartilage surface is cracking, resulting in increased cartilage wear, and the cartilage surface with no amorphous layer is broken, so wear particles calcium and phosphorus content increased rapidly.

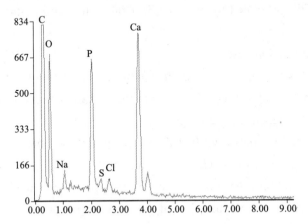

Figure 5-10   EDX Analysis of Wear Particles

5.6   Friction Mechanism Analysis of Reciprocating Rotary Motion

(1) Impact of Load

The contact between the cartilage and the ceramic ball head in the test belongs to the contact between the ball and the surface. According to the Hertz contact principle, their contact area will be a contact circle centered on the contact center, and the contact pressure is elliptical. According to Hertz analysis, the contact radius is

$$r = \sqrt[3]{\frac{3PR\left(\frac{1-v_1^2}{E_1} + \frac{1-v_2^2}{E_2}\right)}{4}}, \tag{5-1}$$

where the equivalent curvature or compound curvature is

$$\frac{1}{R} = \frac{1}{R_1} = \frac{1}{R_2}. \tag{5-2}$$

Ceramic ball radius is R_1, cartilage surface radius is R_2, and the load is P.

Cartilage is a porous aqueous material that is easily deformed after being loaded, and the depth of deformation of the cartilage surface is

$$\frac{1}{R} = \frac{1}{R_1} = \frac{1}{R_2}.$$

(5-3)

It can be seen from the above formula that the contact radius and the surface deformation depth will become larger when the load is increased in the test. With the result that the ceramic ball head cartilage and the contact area become large, the stress concentration which would reduce the contact surface and the deformation of the cartilage surface will be smoother. The roughness is reduced cartilage contact surface, which can lead to soft bone and ceramic balls. The coefficient of friction between the heads is reduced.

(2) The Effect of Speed and Lubrication

When the cartilage surface is in contact with the surface of the ceramic ball head, since both surfaces have a certain roughness, that is, the surface is composed of many different shapes of micro convex peaks and valleys, the actual contact occurs only in a small part of the nominal contact area. The two surfaces of the friction pair always have the interaction of peaks and valleys during the reciprocating friction process. During the interaction process, the higher peaks are prone to elastic deformation until they are flattened, and the lower peaks only elasticize deformation. Due to the large contact stress in the reciprocating friction mode of the point contact, the increase of the speed will aggravate the destruction process of the cartilage surface, which leads to the loss of the two-phase performance of the PVA hydrogel and increases the roughness of the contact surface. The results table is now an increased friction coefficient. Besides, in the reciprocating friction test of cartilage and ceramic ball head, the lubrication of the HA solution also serves to effectively reduce the friction coefficient of the friction pair.

(3) Wear

From the test results, cartilage and ceramic ball head in rubs have two kinds of surface wear embodiment including abrasive wear and fatigue wear, and stainless steel and the wear of the cartilage pair are in the same manner. In the friction pair composed of cartilage and ceramic ball head, the elastic modulus of the ceramic ball head is much larger than the elastic modulus of the cartilage. As the test progresses, the solid phase load in the cartilage gradually increases, and the stress between the microprotrusions on the surface of the friction pair gradually increases. When the micro-convex body forms a favorable angle of attack with the surface of the ceramic ball head, micro-cutting occurs under the action of shearing force to form wear debris. When the microprotrusion forms an unfavorable angle of attack with the surface of the ceramic ball head, the surface will be greatly deformed, and at the same time, under the action of the furrows of the microprotrusions, the material on the surface of the cartilage can be easily worn away. Likewise, under stress reciprocal rotation cycle, when cartilage deformation reaches a certain level the surface, it will crack and eventually lead to fatigue wear surface of the cartilage.

5.7　Summary

In this chapter, the tests use conventional artificial joint cartilage material and a new artificial joint of polyethylene hydrogel in reciprocal rotation and reciprocation testing, provide the basis for the study of cartilage friction mechanism, and explain how to further improve artificial cartilage material.

For the requirements of the friction test of cartilage materials, the existing reciprocating friction tester is modified. The modified testing machine can measure the frictional force in both directions of reciprocating motion, maintain the lubrication environment required by biological materials, realize the dual-purpose of one machine, and perform the reciprocating linear motion friction test and the reciprocating rotary motion friction test.

The reciprocating linear motion friction test and the reciprocating rotary motion friction test were carried out using the established dual-purpose friction tester. The reciprocating linear motion test uses two pairs of cartilage and stainless steel and cartilage and PVA hydrogel artificial cartilage. As the carrier increases the speed of charge, the friction coefficient will be decreased, mainly due to the cartilage surface morphology and deformation. Wear of the cartilage surface is mainly abrasive wear and fatigue wear. The particle size is mainly concentrated between 0 and 4 micrometers, and the number of small-sized abrasive grains is large.

For the friction pair of cartilage and PVA hydrogel, the friction coefficient decreases with the increase of load, and the increase of speed will lead to an increase of friction coefficient. The change of friction coefficient is affected by the surface morphology of cartilage and PVA hydrogel. There are mainly two kinds of wear modes including adhesive wear and surface fatigue wear, which is manifested by PVA hydrogel adhesion on the cartilage surface.

　　A dual reciprocating friction tester has already been established. The friction test is conducted for the hip joint and a ceramic ball head cartilage. The results show that the friction coefficient decreases with the increase of the load in the test, and the friction coefficient increases with the increase of the speed. The wear form is the wear mode of abrasive wear and surface fatigue wear. All test results indicate that HA solution as a lubricant can reduce friction.

Chapter 6
Friction Behavior of Cartilage Under Dynamic Load

6.1 Introduction

In natural human joints, the hip and knee joints are subjected to loads during movement, and the load changes are always dynamic (Unsworth, 1995). For human knee joints, in a gait cycle, after the heel touches the ground, the reaction force of the joint is immediately 2 to 3 times the weight; the peak value of the joint reaction force occurs during the late standing phase, when the toe is about to leave the ground, and then approximately 3 to 4 times the body weight is applied to the human body; at the late phase of the swing phase, the joint reaction force is approximately equal to the body weight; during the entire gait cycle, the joint reaction force of the knee joint moves from the lateral tibial plateau to the medial side. For human hip joints, there are two peaks of joint reaction force during the gait cycle. One peak occurs when the heel touches the ground and reaches 4 times the weight. The other peak occurs before the toes reach the ground and the weight. When the foot is flattened, the joint reaction force is reduced to less than 2 times the body weight. The extensor muscle contracts during the swing phase and the contraction of the extensor muscle cause the thigh to decelerate. At this time, the joint reaction force is less than the body weight. Therefore, it is necessary to study the friction properties of articular cartilage under dynamic loading. In this chapter, the friction properties of cartilage and stainless steel, cartilage and PVA hydrogel, and cartilage and cartilage friction pairs are compared using constant load method and two dynamic load methods. In addition, the effect of roughness on friction is also studied. The friction properties of human cartilage and bovine cartilage were compared.

6.2   Dynamic Load Test of Cartilage

6.2.1   Test Method

(1) Sample Preparation

Three friction pairs are used in this test, including cartilage and cartilage, cartilage and stainless steel, and cartilage and PVA hydrogel. The common sample processing method is used. The samples obtained by sawing and drilling in the experiment are human knee joint cartilage and PVA hydrogel. The PVA hydrogel is obtained by chemical crosslinking method, PVA is dissolved in 80% DMSO aqueous solution, and 15% by weight solution is obtained by freezing and thawing the solution. Cartilage pins have a diameter of about 9 mm, and cartilage pieces have a width of about 11 mm and a length of about 20 mm. The stainless steel material is medical stainless steel, model 317 L; the surface roughness is $Ra = 0.05$, and the medical stainless steel was measured before the experiment.

(2) Test Equipment

The test equipment is the UMT-2 multifunctional friction and wear tester, and the equipment is produced by the American CETR company. The testing machine can achieve accurate dynamic loading through a closed-loop servo system, and the minimum force can reach 0.1 mN. The testing machine can perform micro-tribological and mechanical testing of various materials and lubricants, and can simultaneously measure a variety of signals in situ, such as load, friction, torque, contact resistance, and longitudinal displacement. According to the test requirements, a special fixture is designed to connect with the cartilage pin before the experiment; cartilage pieces, PVA hydrogel and stainless steel are pasted at the bottom of the sample tank. The clamp on which the cartilage pin is mounted on the upper part of the testing machine is connected to the force sensor.

(3) Test Steps

The reciprocating stroke of the cartilage pin sample used in the test was 4 mm, and the reciprocating speed was 2 mm/s. The load in the test is of two types: constant load and dynamic load (see Figure 6-1). The test includes three test methods, a constant load test, a one-minute stand test, and a cyclic load test. In the constant load test, the friction pair maintains a constant load of 25 N. Under the load, the friction is continuously reciprocated for 60 minutes. In the one-minute stand test, the friction pair is unloaded to 0.5 N after the end of the constant load test for 60 minutes. The cartilage pin keeps it still for 1 minute, reloads it to 25 N, and then performs the reciprocating friction test for 30 minutes. In the cyclic load test, the load is cyclic variable load. The load change step in one cycle is as follows: First, a 25 N load is applied to the friction pair, and the load is maintained for 1 second. Then, the cartilage pin moves at a speed of 2 mm/s, that is, the cartilage pin advances 4 mm, and then returns to the original position; the load is reduced to 0.5 N and the load remains unchanged for 4 seconds; the cartilage pin remains stationary and then starts the next cycle. In each test method, three different samples are used for testing. The test result is taken as the value of the last cycle of each test. The results of the three groups of samples need to be averaged. The lubricant in the test is Ringer's solution.

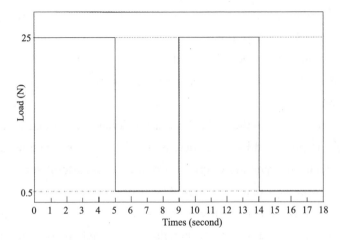

Figure 6-1   Schematic Diagram of Cyclic Load

6.2.2   Friction Between Cartilage and Different Materials

(1) Constant Load Test

The friction coefficients of cartilage and stainless steel, cartilage and PVA hydrogel, and cartilage and cartilage friction pairs were obtained under constant load (see Figure 6-2). In the 60-minute reciprocating friction test, the friction coefficient of cartilage and cartilage friction pairs has not changed, and it remains the lowest among all types of friction pairs. The coefficient of friction fluctuates around 0.025. The friction coefficients of the friction pairs of cartilage and PVA hydrogel and cartilage and stainless steel have kept rising during the experiment. The friction coefficient of the cartilage and stainless steel friction pairs increased faster than that of the cartilage and PVA hydrogel friction pairs. When the test time is 60 minutes, the coefficient of friction between cartilage and stainless steel is 0.266, which is higher than the value of the friction coefficient between cartilage and PVA hydrogel. Under the action of normal saline lubrication and constant load, cartilage and cartilage have the best frictional performance, cartilage and PVA hydrogel have a lower frictional performance, and cartilage and stainless steel have the worst frictional performance.

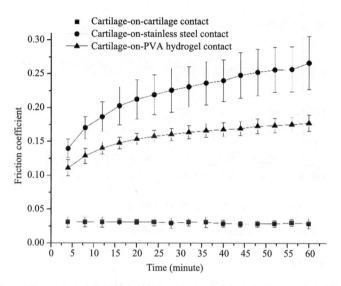

Figure 6-2   Friction Results of Continuous Sliding Tests Under Static Load

(2) Friction Test After Standing for One Minute

The test obtained the reciprocating friction test results of different friction pairs after 1 minute of standing (see Figure 6-3). After keeping it still for one minute while reducing the load to 0.5 N, the friction performance of different friction pairs did not change much in the next 30 minutes of friction test. The friction coefficient of cartilage paired with PVA hydrogel slowly increased in 30 minutes, and the value of the friction coefficient increased from 0.152 to 0.171. The friction coefficient of cartilage paired with stainless steel has always been greater than that of other friction pairs, and the friction coefficient has increased from 0.254 to 0.289. At the same time, it was found that the cartilage-cartilage friction pair can always maintain good friction performance without any increase in friction coefficient.

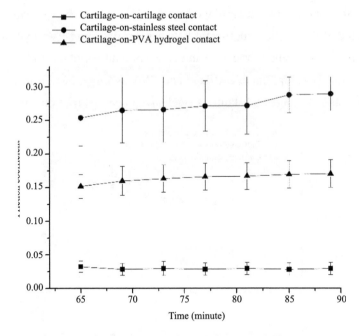

—■— Cartilage-on-cartilage contact
—●— Cartilage-on-stainless steel contact
—▲— Cartilage-on-PVA hydrogel contact

Figure 6-3   Friction Results of One-Minute Load Change Tests

(3) Cyclic Load Test

The change of friction coefficient of three different friction pairs under cyclic load was obtained through experiments (see Figure 6-4). The cartilage-cartilage friction pair maintained the lowest friction coefficient throughout the 60-minute cyclic load test, and the value of the friction coefficient remained unchanged. The friction coefficient of cartilage and stainless steel friction pairs increased rapidly; in the first 20 minutes, the friction coefficient increased from 0.093 to 0.155; after a 40-minute cyclic load friction test, the friction coefficient of cartilage and stainless steel friction pairs reached approximately 0.159, and the value reached relative equilibrium. The friction coefficient of cartilage and PVA hydrogel friction pairs is different from that of cartilage and stainless steel friction pairs, and their growth is relatively slow. In the first 20 minutes, the coefficient of friction between cartilage and PVA hydrogel slowly increased from 0.046 to 0.058, and the coefficient of friction remained small during the rest of the time.

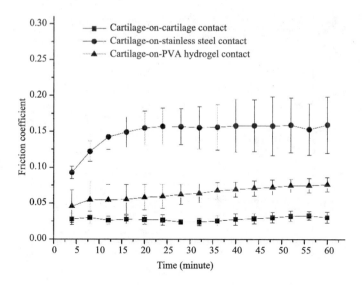

Figure 6-4   Friction Results of Cyclic Load Tests

(4) Comparison of the Results of the Constant Load Test and the Cyclic Load Test

It can be seen from the comparison of the results that the cartilage and cartilage friction pair has always maintained good friction performance, the friction coefficient is about 0.029, and the friction coefficient has not changed at all (see Figure 6-5). The value of the cartilage-to-cartilage friction coefficient is always much smaller than the other two friction pairs. The change of friction coefficient of cartilage and stainless steel friction pair under two load conditions is given in the test. Under constant and cyclic loading, the friction coefficient between cartilage and stainless steel has maintained a large increase. Under cyclic loading, the friction coefficient of the cartilage-stainless steel friction pair is significantly lower than under constant load; at 60 minutes, the friction coefficient is reduced from 0.266 under constant load to 0.159 under cyclic load; it can be seen that the cyclic load test conditions can effectively improve the friction between cartilage and stainless steel. The friction coefficient changes of cartilage and PVA hydrogel under two loading conditions were also obtained in the test. Under cyclic loading, the friction coefficient between cartilage and PVA hydrogel increased slowly and kept low. At 60 minutes, the coefficient of friction between cartilage and PVA hydrogel under cyclic loading decreased from 0.178 to 0.076 under constant load.

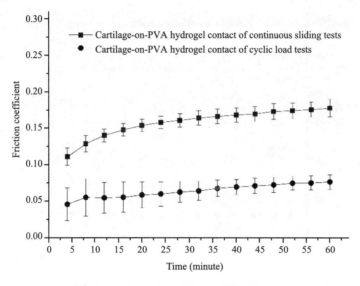

Figure 6-5　Comparison of Cartilage-on-PVA Hydrogel Contact

(5) Comparison of Constant Load Test and One-Minute Standstill Test

　　The test obtained the results of the constant load test and the one-minute test (see Figure 6-6). After the constant load test was performed for 60 minutes, the friction pair started to stand for one minute. During the one-minute standstill of the friction pair, the load was reduced from 25 N to 0.5 N. At the same time, the friction coefficient between cartilage and stainless steel changed. The friction coefficient of the gel friction pair also changed, and the friction coefficient of the cartilage and cartilage friction pair remained unchanged. In the test, the change of friction coefficient was obtained at 4 minutes in different tests. The friction coefficient of cartilage and stainless steel friction pair decreased from 0.266 to 0.254, the friction coefficient of cartilage and PVA hydrogel friction pair decreased from 0.178 to 0.152, and the reduction of cartilage and PVA hydrogel was the largest. At the same time, it can be found that the friction performance of cartilage and stainless steel and cartilage and PVA hydrogel friction pairs cannot be restored to the level before the constant load test after 1 minute of rest and unloading.

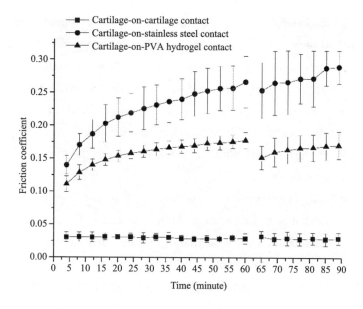

Figure 6-6   Comparison of Continuous Sliding Tests and One-Minute Load Change Tests

6.2.3   Analysis of Friction Mechanism of Cartilage Under Dynamic Load

Cartilage is a two-phase material with good friction properties. The friction performance is related to the boundary lubricant on the surface of cartilage, and the friction performance is also directly related to the liquid and solid phases inside the cartilage. Soltz & Ateshian (1998) used special compression devices and liquid pressure sensors to measure the liquid phase pressure value of the cartilage under compressive load; it was found that the load supported by the liquid phase was close to 100% at the beginning of compression; as time increased, the phase-supported load gradually decreased. Pawaskar, Jin & Fisher (2007) established a model of the frictional movement of metal plates on the surface of cartilage in ABAQUS, and found that as the friction time increased, the load carried by the liquid phase in the cartilage gradually decreased, and the load carried by the solid phase gradually increased.

At the beginning of the reciprocating friction test, the liquid phase in the cartilage bears most of the load on the cartilage in the form of interstitial hydraulic pressure. At the same time, the solid phase matrix only bears a small part of the load. The main source of friction is the relative sliding between the solid phases. The influence of the viscous shear stress between the liquid phase and the liquid phase is negligible; with the extension of the load application time, the liquid phase in the load zone continues to drain, causing the gap hydraulic pressure to decrease, so the solid phase load continues to rise. This will lead to an increase in the coefficient of friction. During the two-phase loading, the proteins and lipids contained in the amorphous layer of the cartilage surface can act as a friction boundary lubricant.

In all tests, the coefficient of friction between cartilage and cartilage has been kept low, although the cartilage pin specimen always bears the load and reciprocates, and the contact position of the cartilage slice specimen in the test is always changing, which is beneficial. The maintenance and recovery of cartilage fluid bearing will facilitate the maintenance of low friction. At the same time, the boundary lubrication component of the surface of the cartilage pin and cartilage sheet also helps to maintain a low coefficient of friction.

Stainless steel is a hard material with only a solid phase. In the reciprocating friction test of cartilage pins and stainless steel pieces, the friction coefficient between cartilage and stainless steel has been increasing, which is related to the decline of the two-phase performance of cartilage. During the continuous reciprocating contact between cartilage and stainless steel, the liquid components in cartilage are continuously lost under the load, the liquid phase load decreases, and the solid phase load increases, which will cause the friction coefficient to increase. In the dynamic load test, the friction coefficient of cartilage and stainless steel decreased at the same time, because during dynamic loading, the cartilage could bear a load of 0.5 N almost half of the time, which was conducive to the partial recovery of the liquid phase in the cartilage and this reduced the friction for subsequent movements.

PVA hydrogel is a typical two-phase material, which has a porous network structure rich in a large amount of liquid phase. PVA hydrogel has a two-phase bearing mechanism similar to cartilage during the process of reciprocating friction with cartilage. At the beginning of friction, the liquid phase component in the PVA hydrogel is subjected to a large number of test loads. As the liquid phase component is continuously lost during the test, the solid phase component load is increased and the friction coefficient is increased. The surface damage of PVA hydrogel will further reduce its two-phase bearing capacity, leading to an increase in friction coefficient. PVA hydrogel has low yield strength and hardness. Under the load stress, PVA hydrogel at the contact points is first in the stage of elastic deformation. As time increases, PVA hydrogel at the contact points will further undergo plastic flow. It will cause damage to the surface of the PVA hydrogel, and the PVA hydrogel material peeled off will cause adhesion between the cartilage and the PVA hydrogel. As the load increases, the elastic deformation of the PVA hydrogel further increases, and the plastic flow of the PVA hydrogel at the contact point will occur faster and more severely, which accelerates the surface damage of the PVA hydrogel and the friction interface. The intensification of surface damage leads to the acceleration of the loss of liquid-phase carrying capacity in PVA hydrogel, and the consequence of the solid-phase component loading in PVA hydrogel is the rising of the friction coefficient.

From the comparison of constant load and cyclic load tests, it can be found that under cyclic load, the coefficient of friction between PVA hydrogel and cartilage has been kept at a low level, which is the result of the continuous recovery of the two-phase bearing capacity of PVA hydrogel. Compared with the cartilage-to-cartilage friction test results, it can be seen that the two-phase bearing capacity of PVA hydrogel is not as effective as cartilage, which is related to the PVA hydrogel's modulus, porosity, and porous structure composition. Moreover, the surface of the PVA hydrogel lacks a boundary lubricant enrichment layer similar to the amorphous layer on the cartilage surface, which will affect the friction properties of the PVA hydrogel.

Forster & Fisher (1999) studied the one-minute unloading test of cartilage pins and stainless steel; in the test, they found that after one minute of complete unloading, the friction coefficient between cartilage and stainless steel decreased significantly. In this test, not only the cartilage pin was paired with stainless steel, but also the cartilage and cartilage and the cartilage and PVA hydrogel were tested. The results showed that after one minute of unloading, the friction coefficient between cartilage pins and PVA hydrogel decreased most obviously, which indicated that the PVA hydrogel part was suitable as a substitute for natural cartilage.

6.3   Effect of Material Surface Roughness on Cartilage Friction Properties

6.3.1   Test Method

In this test, the friction properties between the cartilage pin sample and medical stainless steel 317 L with different roughness were tested. For the test, 9 mm diameter bovine joint cartilage pin samples and medical stainless steel were used as friction pairs. There are three types of medical stainless steel samples, including three types of surface roughness *Ra* values, namely 0.05 microns, 0.5 microns and 0.8 microns. The test equipment is UMT-3 multifunctional friction and abrasion tester, produced by the American CETR company. In the test, the cartilage pin sample had a reciprocating stroke of 4 mm, a reciprocating speed of 2 mm/s, a load of 25 N, and a lubricating solution of physiological saline. The cartilage pin was continuously reciprocated for 5 minutes during the entire test, and the friction coefficient within 5 minutes was compared. Each test method uses two sets of samples for testing, and the test results are the averaged value.

6.3.2 Influence of Roughness on Friction Performance

The test has obtained the effect of roughness on the cartilage friction performance (see Figure 6-7). The surface roughness of stainless steel samples has a certain effect on the friction properties of cartilage. The lower the surface roughness of stainless steel samples, the smaller the coefficient of friction between friction samples. The strength of articular cartilage is much lower than that of stainless steel; under the action of load, the uneven surface of stainless steel is prone to cause plastic deformation and furrows on the surface of cartilage, thereby increasing the coefficient of friction. The rough stainless steel surface has more sharp peaks, and the cartilage has a relatively soft surface. The load on the contact surface of the cartilage and stainless steel causes these peaks to be embedded in the cartilage surface. During the reciprocating friction process, the amorphous layer of the cartilage surface will be scratched by the convex peak, and then it is lost. This will reduce the boundary lubricant of the cartilage and stainless steel contact surface and increase the permeability of the cartilage surface. The decrease in the carrying capacity of the middle and liquid phases will inevitably increase the friction coefficient between cartilage and stainless steel. For relatively rough stainless steel, that is, 0.5 micron and 0.8 micron stainless steel, the friction coefficient between them and the cartilage is similar, but there is a certain gap with the low friction coefficient of 0.05 micron stainless steel.

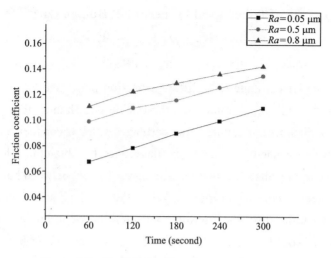

Figure 6-7   The Effect of Roughness on the Friction

6.4   Comparison of Tribological Properties of Human Cartilage and Bovine Cartilage

6.4.1   Test Method

In this test, the differences in tribological properties of human cartilage and bovine cartilage were tested. The study included three matching methods: cartilage and stainless steel, cartilage and PVA hydrogel, and cartilage and cartilage. The test used multiple human cartilage pins and bovine cartilage pins with a diameter of 9 mm. The PVA hydrogel was prepared by a chemical crosslinking method. PVA was dissolved in 80% DMSO to obtain an aqueous solution, and the solution mass fraction was 15% by weight. The solution was frozen and thawed to obtain a sample. The stainless steel material was 317 L medical stainless steel, and the surface roughness Ra was 0.05 micrometer. The test equipment was UMT-3 multifunctional friction and wear tester, which was produced by the American CETR company. In the test, the cartilage pin sample had a reciprocating stroke of 4 mm, a reciprocating speed of 2 mm/s, a load of 25 N, and a lubricating solution of physiological saline. In the test, the cartilage pin sample had a reciprocating stroke of 4 mm, a reciprocating speed of 2 mm/s, a load of 25 N, and a lubricating solution of physiological saline. Each friction pair was tested three times in the test, and the average value of the friction coefficient was taken. The test time for each test was 5 minutes.

6.4.2 Comparison of Tribological Properties of Human Cartilage and Bovine Cartilage

The test results show the friction characteristics of human articular cartilage and bovine articular cartilage with different friction pairs (see Figure 6-8). It has been found in the existing literature that the thickness of human femur cartilage is greater than the thickness of bovine femur cartilage, which is conducive to increasing the liquid-carrying capacity of human cartilage, thereby obtaining a lower friction coefficient. The test results show that the friction coefficient between human cartilage and stainless steel is not much different. When the cartilage and stainless steel are subjected to a friction test, the friction coefficient between human cartilage and stainless steel is slightly higher than that of the corresponding bovine cartilage stainless steel pair. When cartilage is paired with PVA hydrogel and cartilage, the friction coefficient obtained by human cartilage in the test is low.

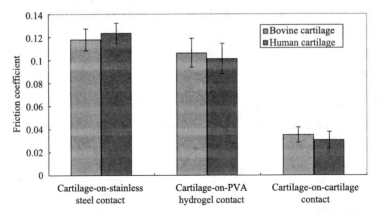

Figure 6-8   Comparison of Frictional Properties of Human Cartilage and Bovine Cartilage

6.5 Summary

UMT series micro friction testing machine was used for the reciprocating friction test of cartilage and cartilage, cartilage and stainless steel, and cartilage and PVA hydrogel. The test load is a constant and dynamic load, including three test methods, namely a constant load test, a one-minute stand test, and a cyclic load test. In all tests, the cartilage-cartilage friction pair always maintained good friction performance, with a friction coefficient of about 0.029. There was no change in the friction coefficient during the test. Under cyclic loading, the friction coefficient of the cartilage and stainless steel friction pair is significantly lower than under constant load; the friction performance of cartilage and PVA hydrogel is greatly improved, and the value of the friction coefficient is one-third of the value under constant load. In the one-minute test, the friction properties of the cartilage and stainless steel and the cartilage and PVA hydrogel friction pairs could not be recovered, and the friction coefficient was difficult to reach the value of the constant load test; the friction performance of cartilage and PVA hydrogel recovered fastest.

The test uses cartilage paired with stainless steel to study the effect of stainless steel surface roughness on the cartilage friction properties. The results show that the surface roughness of stainless steel samples has a certain effect on the friction properties of cartilage. The lower the surface roughness of stainless steel samples, the smaller the coefficient of friction between the friction samples.

The cartilage and stainless steel, cartilage and PVA hydrogel, and cartilage and cartilage pairs were used to study the tribological properties of human cartilage and bovine cartilage. The results show that the friction coefficient between human cartilage and stainless steel is not much different. At the same time, the friction coefficient obtained by human cartilage is lower in the test.

Chapter 7
Tribological Behavior of Articular Cartilage in Compound Movement

7.1 Introduction

Natural knee joints have complex movement modes. The goal of artificial knee joints is to achieve a variety of movement modes of natural human knee joints. After the patient received the joint replacement, there were multiple sets of frictional contact surfaces in the artificial knee joint, such as the interface between the femoral condyle and the artificial meniscus, the interface between the artificial meniscus and the artificial tibia, and the interface between the artificial tibia and the lower tibia. In the daily use of artificial joints, friction exists on these interfaces, which will cause different degrees of wear after prolonged use; for example, UHMWPE prostheses in artificial knee joint prostheses will wear. When the wear is more serious, the surface of the artificial joint will be worn. Many abrasive particles are generated. The particles cause osteolysis in patients implanted with artificial knee joints; friction can cause serious problems such as artificial joint destruction and loosening, and lead to failure of joint replacement surgery in the late stage. Therefore, before artificial joints are used in the clinic, testers need to perform various experimental evaluations of artificial joints. There are many types of tribological performance evaluation tests for joint materials, which are mainly divided into two parts: the conventional tribology test and the joint simulation exercise test. The conventional tests of joint materials are mainly carried out on various types of friction and wear testing machines. The friction and wear tests are performed by contact methods such as sliding and rolling. This is the simplest and most effective way to evaluate the friction and wear performance of materials. For articular cartilage materials, due to the complex multi-degree-of-

116

freedom motion mode of the knee joint, it is not enough to use conventional test methods to test the friction and wear performance. It is also necessary to use a testing machine that mimics various types of motion of the natural knee joint.

7.2   Knee Movement

Natural knee joints have complex movements, which are roughly divided into six movements, three of which are rotations: interior-exterior, flexion-extension, and varus-valgus; three movements are displacements: anterior-posterior translation, medial-lateral translation and axial load. As can be seen from the result, the six types of movement of the knee joint are interrelated. The tibiofemoral joint also undergoes internal or external rotation while flexing or straightening, and the femoral tibia undergoes front-to-back displacement and medial and lateral movement. Displacement, longitudinal separation and squeezing are directly related to the allocation of the standing phase and the oscillating phase during the body's movement. In daily life, the flexion and extension of the knee joint are $0°-117°$, the range of internal rotation and external rotation is $4°-5°$, the flexion and extension range during walking is $0°-70°$, and the flexion and extension range of downstairs is $0°-90°$. When people sit down, the range is form $0°-93°$. The movement of the knee joint from the straight position to $20°$ flexion is rolling, and from $20°$ flexion to full flexion, it is mainly sliding with a small amount of rolling. The result shows the knee load changes in the human body during walking. As shown in the result, when a person is walking, the load between the femur and tibia is much greater than the body weight, and it can reach 4.3 times the bodyweight under fast walking conditions.

7.3   Standards and Classification of Artificial Knee Joint Simulation Testing Machine

7.3.1   Application of Simulation Testing Machine

The tribological performance evaluation of the artificial knee joint is usually divided into two parts: the conventional tribology test and the joint simulated exercise test. The conventional tests of artificial knee joints are mainly carried out in sliding contact on various types of pin-disk friction and wear testing machines, which is the simplest and most effective way to evaluate the friction and wear performance of materials. For the artificial knee joint, because of its complex multi-degree-of-freedom motion mode, the conventional test method is not enough to test its friction and wear performance, and it needs to be tested using friction and wear tests that mimic the various modes of motion of the natural knee joint.

In order to imitate the various movements of the natural knee joint, a special artificial knee joint simulation test bench needs to be developed. The artificial knee joint simulation test bench should simulate the various movements and forces of the knee joint as much as possible to verify whether the geometry and the structure of the artificial knee joint can meet the needs of patients after surgical replacement. On the artificial knee joint simulation test bench, it is necessary to pass a long-term large-cycle test to detect the friction and wear performance of the artificial knee joint and predict the life of the entire joint. Ungethum & Stallforth (1977) and others believe that the joint simulation test bench must meet the following conditions:

(1) Its rotary motion mode can provide extension, flexion, and internal, external and axial movement;

(2) Its range of motion can be adjusted steplessly, and the applied load has a cyclic form of double peaks;

(3) The maximum and minimum values of its load need to be continuously adjustable to simulate different types of gait and different weights;

(4) Its pace is continuously adjustable;

(5) It can be used to test current commercial joint prostheses without pretreatment;

(6) It is temperature-controllable lubricating medium, filtering of abrasive particles for analysis;

(7) It can measure friction torque, deformation, loading, damping and temperature of the prosthetic sliding surface.

Researchers have developed various types of artificial knee joint test benches that have been able to meet most of the requirements mentioned by Ungethum & Stallforth (1977). At present, there are three main types: spherical contact type, prosthetic force and motion direct control type, and the other is the knee muscle force reconstruction type. The spherical contact type is the pairing of the artificial knee joint material ball with the artificial tibial material platform, and sometimes the disc surface contacts the platform to obtain the friction and wear performance in the multi-degree-of-freedom motion mode of the knee joint, especially when the spherical structure is matched. Direct control of prosthetic force and motion can be used for clinical prosthesis testing. It has the largest number and is most widely used. It can control the displacement and force of the prosthesis and can achieve the goal of simulating human knee joint movement. The knee muscle force reconstruction type uses a cylinder or a motor to drive the device to simulate the muscle force effects of the knee quadriceps and can reconstruct the patellofemoral and tibiofemoral joints to realize knee force and motion simulation. Researchers use different methods for different types of testing machines. Spherical contact knee joint simulation testing machine is mainly used to study the friction and wear performance of modified prosthetic materials; knee joint muscle force reconstruction type and prosthetic force and motion direct control type are more widely used. They can be used for different types of prostheses designed to study friction and wear performance, to study the movement mode closely related to the friction and wear performance of artificial knee joint prosthesis, and to study the surface and internal stress distribution of the artificial joint. The artificial knee joint simulation testing machine for direct control of prosthetic force and motion can be regulated by the three standards of the above-mentioned International Organization for Standardization, and many researchers and some companies have also started testing according to these three standards. The spherical contact type and knee muscle force reconstruction type knee joint simulation testing machine does not have corresponding ISO standards to follow. At present, researchers only design for their research purposes.

7.3.2   ISO Standard for Knee Joint Simulation Test

At present, the Chinese national standard is knee joint prosthesis standard YY 0502-2005, which regulates knee joint prostheses. There is no standard for the artificial knee joint simulation test. The ISO has artificial knee simulator test standards, which include three parts:

(1) ISO14243-1: 2002, Surgical implants—Wear of total knee joint prostheses—Part 1: Loads and load parameters of knee wear-testing machines and related test environmental conditions;

(2) ISO14243-2: 2000, Surgical implants—Wear of total knee prostheses—Part 2: Measurement methods;

(3) ISO14243-3: 2004, Surgical implants—Wear of total knee joint prostheses—Part 3: Load and displacement parameters of knee wear-testing machines and related test environmental conditions.

ISO14243-1: 2002 and ISO14243-3: 2004 both specify similar test speeds and durations as well as test sample shapes and environmental requirements for the test. For specific motion control methods, there is a certain difference between ISO14243-1: 2002 and ISO14243-3: 2004. In the standard, the force or displacement error is controlled within ± 5% of the maximum value, and the time cycle error is controlled within ± 3%. ISO14243-2: 2002 specifies the method for evaluating the wear of artificial knee joints. The basic parameters are as follows: Tribological test frequency is 1 Hz ± 0.1 Hz, the lubricating liquid is 25% ± 2% calf serum deionized water balance solution, and the ambient temperature is maintained at room temperature.

ISO14243-1: 2002 is a simulation standard based on the motion of the knee joint (see Figure 7-1). It specifies the control torque curve of flexion/extension angular motion, axial load, forward and backward displacement force, and internal and external rotation of the tibia, as shown in the result. The ISO14243-3: 2004 is a simulation standard based on knee displacement, which specifies the simulator's axial load, flexion/extension angular motion, anteroposterior displacement, and tibial rotation angle control curves, where the x axis is the motion cycle, and the y axis is the corresponding parameter.

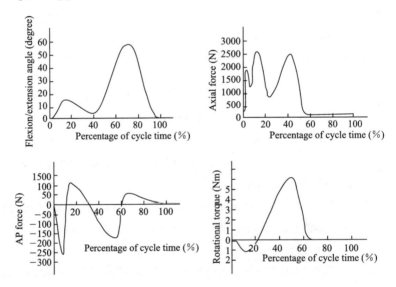

Figure 7-1　Knee Simulation Based on Load Control

7.3.3   Three Types of Testing Machines

(1) Spherical Contact Testing Machine

Spherical contact testing machine is relatively simple to manufacture and maintain, mainly focusing on testing of materials (see Figure 7-2). Wang, Essner, Stark & Dumbleton (1999) used a disc-to-surface contact testing machine to study prosthetic materials. The testing machine is realized by retrofitting the existing reciprocating abrasion testing machine with vertical axis rotation. The disc reciprocates around the horizontal axis at a frequency of 30 Hz. The UHMWPE surface is wound at a frequency of 0 Hz to 90°. The vertical axis performs internal and external rotational movements, with a constant load of 1150 N (15 MPa), and each cycle moves 37.5 mm. Saikko, Ahlroos & Calonius (2001) modified the existing hip joint tester to obtain a spherical contact artificial knee joint simulation tester. The principle and the actual objects are shown in the result. Movement is 5, forward and backward displacement is 5 mm, static vertical loading is 2000 N, gait cycle is 1.08 Hz. Oate, Comin, Braceras, Garcia, Viviente, Brizuela, Garagorri, Peris & Alava (2001) have used a spherical contact knee joint simulation testing machine with UHMWPE. The ball sample was combined with a rolling and sliding motion with a load of 500 N and a frequency of 2 Hz.

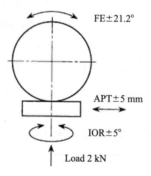

Figure 7-2   Artificial Knee Joint Simulation Test Bench Used by Saikko, Ahlroos & Calonius

(2) Prosthetic Force and Motion Direct Control Testing Machine

Prosthetic force and motion direct control type testing machines are used in the testing of clinical prostheses, the largest number of which is also most widely used. At first, most of these types of testing machines could only imitate one or two kinds of knee joint movements. Such testing machines manufactured in the later stages gradually took the ISO standard as a reference. At the same time, many manufacturers also launched such testing machine products for the ISO standard. Walker & Hsieh (1977) established a testing machine capable of testing 9 prostheses simultaneously for prosthesis testing. The prosthesis achieved 45° flexion and extension and applied 2 times the bodyweight along the axis of the femur. DiAngelo & Harrington (1992) developed a testing machine that can control the axial compressive force and the angle of flexion and straightening, and also used cams to realize the forward and backward displacement curve. The testing machine built by Grood & Suntay (1983) has 6 degrees of freedom, contains 3 kinds of displacements and 3 kinds of rotational movements, has a device that simulates soft tissue, and performs flexion and extension movements around the horizontal axis through the femur. For the flexion and extension movement axis, the forward and backward displacements are performed along the horizontal axis of the eversion movement. The knee joint simulation testing machine used by Desjardins, Walker, Haider & Perry (2000) represents the latest form of the current testing machine. The testing machine includes 4 workbenches, which can be tested simultaneously. Each workbench has 6 degrees of freedom and can operate at a frequency of 50 Hz. The gait frequency is 0.8 Hz; it can test the knee joint prosthesis load, and there are springs and other mechanisms to simulate the impact of soft tissue on the joint; the testing machine can simultaneously measure the specific parameters of various types of artificial knee joint motion.

(3) Knee Joint Muscle Force Reconstruction Type Testing Machine

The friction and wear of the artificial knee joint are related to many factors and mainly affected by the movement pattern and stress changes. The knee joint muscle force reconstruction testing machine uses a cylinder or a motor to drive the device, which can simulate the quadriceps and muscle forces in the lower limbs, the force and movement of the knee joint, and simultaneously the patellofemoral and tibiofemoral joints; therefore, this testing machine is the closest to the real state, and it is of great significance to study the three-dimensional force and motion of the knee joint prosthesis and the effect on the friction and wear of the knee joint. Hersh, Hillberry & Kettelkamp (1981) used hydraulic servo technology to achieve flexion and extension, internal and external rotation and forward and backward movement, and Rovick, Reuben, Schrager & Walker (1991) established a dynamic loading mechanism to achieve three-dimensional motion control. Elias, Kumagai, Mitchell, Mizuno, Mattessich, Webb & Chao (2002) used this type of testing machine to study the effects of fixed and movable bearing prostheses on the motion and wear of artificial knee joints.

Guess & Maletsky (2005) developed a dynamic knee joint simulator, the Kansas Knee Simulator (KKS). The movement is achieved by a hydraulic cylinder controlled by a servo valve, and the position and force on each axis can be measured and controlled. The function of the quadriceps muscles is controlled by hydraulic cylinder simulation to control the knee joint force and movement, as well as the hip flexion angle. A simulation model is also established on the computer to predict the entire process, and then the measured results are compared with the simulation model results to obtain the constraints of the simulation model. The simulation model is used to control the testing machine to achieve movement, and the artificial knee joint is preset in three dimensions with force and movements. The results show that the measured results of the lateral displacement of the artificial joint, the forward and backward displacement, and the tibial plateau rotation angle are in good agreement with the simulation model results. As the flexion angle increases, the errors between the two also increase.

7.3.4   Comparison of Testing Machines

The three types of testing machines have their characteristics, and the testing methods are also different: although the spherical contact type has a simple structure but a narrow range of use, it is suitable for the initial friction and wear performance test of the prosthetic material; the prosthetic force and motion direct control type reconstruction of the tibiofemoral joint are able to perform long-term wear test; knee muscle force reconstruction type is closest to the real joint, completely reconstructing knee joint patellofemoral joint and tibiofemoral joint. It can be used in joint force measurement. In the specific test, a suitable testing machine should be selected according to the purpose of the test. The different points of various types of testing machines can be summarized as shown in Table 7-1.

Table 7-1　Comparison of Artificial Knee Joint Simulation Test Bench

Testing machine	Specimen	Maximum freedom of motion	Joint	Goal	Test
spherical contact type	artificial femoral material ball head and artificial tibial material platform	4	tibiofemoral joint	test the tribological properties of the artificial knee joint prosthesis material	the spherical structure mimics the knee joint motion mode, the structure is simple and easy to implement, and it can perform long-term wear tests
direct control of prosthetic force and motion	prosthetic knee joint prosthesis	6	tibiofemoral joint	test tribological performance of artificial knee prosthesis, the relationship between controlled and uncontrolled motion	direct control of the prosthetic force and motion parameters, long-term Abrasion test
knee muscle force reconstruction	prosthetic knee joint prosthesis	6	patella femoral joint, tibiofemoral joint, tibiofemoral joint	joint mechanical and kinematic testing of artificial knee joint	reconstructing joint muscle force, complex system difficult to perform long-term wear test

7.4　Development of Artificial Knee Joint Simulation Testing Machine

7.4.1　Structural Design

According to the international standard ISO14243-3: 2004, an artificial knee joint simulation exercise testing machine was established. This type of test stand is a displacement control mode. It uses three displacement curves and one load curve to control the movement and force of the knee joint. It simulates the three degrees of freedom of internal and external rotation, flexion and extension, and forward and backward displacement of the human knee joint. It also includes a longitudinal squeeze loading motion and varus motion; the test bench has its temperature control system and lubrication system, which can simulate the temperature and lubrication environment in the human body.

Various motion modes in the testing machine are realized by cam mechanism and connecting rod mechanism, and the longitudinal compression load is applied to the tibial prosthesis by servo electric cylinder; the testing machine also collects the information of the flexion-straightening motion angular displacement of the knee joint movement to extract the angle. The displacement phase information is then used to control the loading time of the electric servo cylinder to ensure that the phase of the load curve is consistent with the displacement curve of the knee joint. The testing machine controls the shape or motion parameters of the cam, timing belt gear train, and linkage mechanism, *etc.*, and can simulate different forms of motion of the knee joint. The testing machine collects the angular displacement information of the knee joint movement through a rotary encoder. The testing machine extracts the angular displacement phase information to control the loading time of the electric servo cylinder to ensure that the phase of the load curve is consistent with the displacement curve of the knee joint. This test bench can collect five parameters, that is, the flexion-straightening angle of the knee prosthesis, the angle of internal and external rotation, forward and backward displacement, forward and backward shear force and axial force. The temperature of the testing machine's lubricating fluid is controlled in PID mode, and it is maintained at a constant temperature of 37 degrees Celsius to simulate the physiological environment of the artificial knee joint. The knee joint test bench is designed with three work stations, which can simultaneously perform three artificial knee joint simulation tests. In the lab, one station is currently installed.

7.4.2   Mechanism

The schematic diagram of the mechanical transmission of the artificial knee joint simulation testing machine is shown (see Figure 7-3). The principle content has been authorized by the invention patent. The main components of this simulation testing machine are as follows: (1) femoral prosthesis, (2) tibial plateau, (3) AP driven rod, (4) servo electric cylinder, (5) AP timing belt wheel train, (6) motor, (7) IE cam, (8) FE cam, (9) IE driven rod system, (10) IE curved disk, (11) FE driven rod system, (12) FE disc, (13) bevel gear pair, (14) IE timing belt train and (15) AP cam. A schematic diagram of the knee joint prosthesis mounting section is shown. The composition of the sample mounting part is as follows: femoral prosthesis, tibial plateau, AP follower rod, IE synchronous belt wheel train, tibial plate holder, bearing, fixed cylinder and servo-electric cylinder loading head.

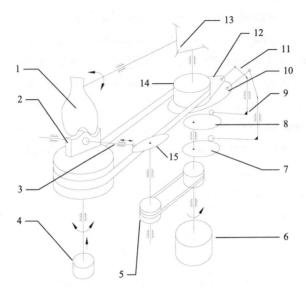

Figure 7-3 Schematic of Transmission

When it is working, the motor drives the AP timing belt wheel train, IE cam and FE cam to rotate. The AP synchronous belt wheel system drives the AP cam to rotate. The AP cam makes the AP follower rod move back and forth. A tibial platform bracket is installed on the AP follower rod. Therefore, the tibial platform in the tibial platform bracket will follow the AP follower rod. The IE cam cooperates with the IE driven rod system to convert the rotation of the IE cam into the IE driven rod system swing, the IE driven rod system is connected with the IE synchronous belt wheel system, and the swing of the IE driven rod system is converted to the IE synchronous belt wheel. The IE synchronous belt wheel train is connected with the tibial platform bracket. The tibial platform bracket drives the tibial platform to realize the reciprocating rotary motion under the support of the bearing and the fixed cylinder. The FE cam is connected with the FE driven rod system, and the rotation of the FE cam is converted into the swing of the FE driven rod system. The FE driven rod system is connected with the bevel gear pair, and the swing of the FE driven rod system is converted into the reciprocation of the bevel gear pair. Rotational movement is achieved. The bevel gear vice shaft end is connected with the femoral prosthesis to achieve the flexion-straightening movement of the femoral prosthesis. The longitudinal compression loading is implemented by a servo-electric cylinder. Specifically, the servo-electric cylinder loading head is applied to the tibia platform to ensure that the phase of the load curve is consistent with the displacement curve of the knee joint.

7.4.3   Motion Parameters

The result shows the comparison of the motion and force curves in the ISO standard with the results in the test. This test bench measures the FE curve of buckling-straightening motion, the IE curve of internal-external rotation, the AP curve of forward-backward movement, and the force-load curve of longitudinal separation and compression. The results are compared with the curves of the ISO14243-3. The results show that the amplitudes and waveforms of the four curves and the standard curve are basically the same, which fits the standard waveform well and meets the requirements of the ISO standard. The IE curve peak value and standard curve are respectively 0.9 degree and 0.53 degree. During the test, LabView was used to monitor the testing machine in real-time. The operation interface of the computer was also developed.

7.5   Test Method

7.5.1   Sample Preparation

The cartilage piece was matched with a 317 L stainless steel cylinder for testing. The cartilage piece sample was 16-25 mm wide, 28-38 mm long, 12-15 mm thick, with stainless steel cylinder diameter 55 mm, thickness 30 mm, and surface roughness 0.5 micron. Using the sample processing method in Chapter 2, the cartilage film samples obtained are human knee joint cartilage film and bovine joint cartilage film. It can be seen that the sample in the sample tank is fixed with model plaster, which is a dental high-strength and low-expansion artificial plaster. It is a super hard plaster produced by Heraeus Gosa Dental Co., Ltd., which is suitable for the precision casting model, fine powder, high curing strength and smooth edges. The curing time of this type of gypsum is 10-13 minutes, and the linear curing expansion is 0.07%.

The specific method of fixing the cartilage slice sample is as follows:

(1) Put gypsum into a bowl for blending according to the water/powder ratio (ml/g): 22:100;

(2) Adjust by hand for 60 seconds, or use a vacuum mixer to select 200-

300 rpm, and reconcile for 30 seconds;

(3) The adjusted slurry is poured into the sample container, and the distance between the surface of the cartilage piece and the bottom surface of the stainless steel cylinder is kept constant during each sample pouring.

(4) After 10 minutes, the gypsum is cured, and the surface of the cured gypsum is cleaned.

7.5.2　Test Equipment

In the observation of the specimen, the overall observation of the specimen was performed using the VHX-600E ultra-depth 3D microscope system and an ESEM to observe the worn specimen. The microscopy system was produced by Japan's KEYENCE. The physical map of the three-dimensional microscope system has a 54 million-pixel CCD, which enables ultra-deep and high-resolution observation. It achieves more than 20 times the depth of field of an optical microscope. It can change the field of view and perform repeated measurements of 1600 × 1200 Pixel high-resolution and 15-inch LCD monitor. The microscopic changes of the samples in the test were observed using ESEM. ESEM is a product of the American FEI company and the model number is XL30. In the observation of abrasive particles, ESEM and AFM are used at the same time. Among them, AFM uses the Nanoscope-III AFM of the American DI Company. In the energy spectrum analysis, the Genesis energy spectrometer provided by ESEM was used for correlation analysis. The particle size analysis of the abrasive particles was performed using an LS13320 laser particle size analyzer, which was produced by Beckman Coulter Inc.

7.5.3　Test Procedure

In the knee joint simulated load test, the specimens were cartilage pieces and 317L stainless steel, and 317L was a cylindrical specimen. This test belongs to the most simplified form of knee joint movement and the line contact form during exercise. If the human body is loaded by the physiological load, the stress will exceed the stress range of the human joint. Therefore, a constant load loading method is used in the test. The specific test steps are as follows:

(1) A light load 640 N test was performed with bovine articular cartilage, and a simulated exercise test with a heavy load of 1000 N was also performed. At this time, the frictional contact stress reached about 2.5 MPa and 3.5 MPa respectively, and the

test time was 1 hour. Then, after 1 hour the cartilage wear and surface morphology changed, and the wear conditions under different loads were compared; among them, the test under 1000 N load was also performed on the sample with the observation at 20 min to understand the process of cartilage wear.

(2) The human joint cartilage was used to perform a simulated exercise test at a load of 1000 N. The test time was 1 hour. The cartilage wear status and surface morphology changes after 1 hour were observed, and it was compared with the bovine joint cartilage wear test.

(3) In the test, the exercise mode included flexion and extension movement of the knee joint, forward and backward displacement movement, and internal and external rotation movement. The axial load was constant. Each type of test was performed twice, and the gait frequency in the test was 0.5 Hz.

7.6   Friction and Wear of Articular Cartilage Under Combined Motion

7.6.1   Force and Motion Curves

In this test, a knee joint simulated exercise testing machine is used to perform the test, and the movement can be detected in real time. Various sports state curves are obtained and based on the sensors on the testing machine.

7.6.2   Bovine Cartilage/Stainless Steel for One Hour

In the test, bovine cartilage and stainless steel are sample materials, the load is 640 N, and the test results are obtained after one hour of frictional movement. The result shows the topography of the cartilage surface under the microscope and the measurement of cartilage surface wear scars. As can be seen from the result (see Figure 7-4 before contents), the wear scar on the surface of the cartilage is wide and narrow in the shape of an inverted triangle. Through multi-point measurement, the wear scar depth after calculation is 130.2 ± 56.1 microns, and the wear scar width is 404.3 ± 57.3 microns. It shows an enlarged view of the corresponding positions of cartilage surface wear marks and three-dimensional topography. As a result, there are many wear marks on the surface of cartilage, and the direction of the wear marks is along the direction of the line of contact between the cartilage and the stainless steel cylinder. Because the cartilage surface is in linear contact with stainless steel, and the surface stress of the two in line contact is concentrated, the wear marks on the cartilage surface produced in the test are the result of stress concentration.

7.6.3   Bovine Cartilage/Stainless Steel Heavy Load Exercise for 20 Minutes

The test results of bovine cartilage and stainless steel after moving for 20 minutes under 1000 N load are shown in the results (see Figure 7-5 before contents). It shows the topography of the cartilage surface under a microscope. The result shows the measurement of cartilage surface wear scars. The result shows an enlarged view and three-dimensional topography of the corresponding positions of cartilage surface wear marks. It can be seen that there are a few wear marks on the surface of the cartilage, and the direction of the wear marks is along the direction of the contact line between the cartilage and the stainless steel cylinder. The multi-point measurement shows that the wear scar depth is 69.6 ± 35.5 microns, and the wear scar width is 355.9 ± 68.9 microns.

7.6.4   Bovine Cartilage/Stainless Steel Heavy Load Exercise for One Hour

The cartilage surfaces of cattle cartilage and stainless steel after grinding for one hour under a load of 1000 N are shown in the result (see Figure 7-6 before contents). It shows the topography of the cartilage surface under a microscope. It shows the measurement of cartilage surface wear scars. It shows an enlarged view and three-dimensional topography of the corresponding positions of cartilage surface wear marks. It can be seen that large damaged holes appear on the surface of the cartilage, the cartilage layer of the holes has been stripped, and the subchondral bone has been exposed. The multi-point measurement shows that the depth of the wear scar reaches 438.8 ± 51.8 microns, and the maximum diameter of the surface damage is close to 1 mm, with a range of 737.1 ± 232.5 microns.

7.6.5   Human Cartilage/Stainless Steel Heavy Load Exercise for One Hour

The cartilage surface morphology of human cartilage and stainless steel column samples after abrasion at 1000 N for one hour is examined. It shows the measurement of cartilage surface wear scars. The results include an enlarged view and three-dimensional topography of the corresponding positions of cartilage surface wear marks. There are several obvious wear scars on the surface of the cartilage. The depth of the wear scars is 499.1 ± 90.2 microns, and the width of the wear scars is 675.1 ± 54.1 microns.

7.6.6   ESEM Observation and Elemental Analysis

(1) Beef Cartilage/Stainless Steel Heavy Load Exercise for 20 Minutes

The results show the morphological observation of the cartilage surface under ESEM after the simulated movement of bovine cartilage and stainless steel under a load of 1000 N for 20 minutes (see Figure 7-7). It can be found that there are a large number of strip-shaped wear scars on the surface of the cartilage with a width of more than 100 micrometers. The unworn surface of the cartilage in the tests shows that there are a few particles on the surface of the cartilage. The energy spectrum analysis was also used in the same position. From the energy spectrum analysis chart, it can be found that there is no change in the composition of the cartilage surface elements.

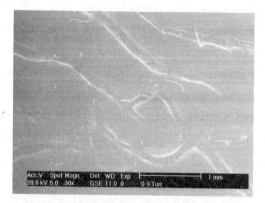

Figure 7-7   ESEM Image of Cartilage Surface

The results show the observation diagrams and energy spectrum analysis results of cartilage surface wear scars. It can be seen that the bottom surface of the wear scar is relatively flat, and a small number of particles are scattered. The elemental analysis of the bottom surface can measure that the iron content reaches 0.24% by weight. Because the material that rubs against cartilage is stainless steel, it can be found that the iron element of the cartilage wear surface mainly comes from the transfer of stainless steel cylindrical material to the surface of cartilage during the friction process.

(2) Beef Cartilage/Stainless Steel of Heavy Load Exercise for One Hour

The result shows the surface observation of bovine cartilage and stainless steel after one hour of movement under a load of 1000 N. It can be seen that there are large defects on the surface of the cartilage. It can be found that the fibrous tissue of the cartilage section is exposed, and it can be seen that the surface structure of the broken surface is uncovered. The results of EDX elemental analysis of the cartilage damaged on the surface are examined. The surface calcium content reached 14.76% by weight and phosphorus content reached 6.65% by weight, which also contained 0.52% by weight iron. It can be seen that the content of calcium and phosphorus increased significantly, indicating that the cartilage in the calcification area had been revealed, and the lamellar structure of cartilage had been severely damaged.

The result is an observation diagram of the abrasive particles on the surface of the cartilage. There are also the results of the EDX elemental analysis of cartilage surface abrasive particles. It can be seen that there are a large number of wear particles on the surface of cartilage, the shape of the particles distributed on the surface varies, and the shapes of the wear particles are round, which are in a long and irregular shape. By analyzing the EDX element of the particles, it can be known that part of the particle element contains iron and chromium, for example, the particle at Position 1 contains 0.26% by weight chromium and 1.26% by weight iron; the elemental composition of the particles of the cartilage surface is consistent in composition and does not contain chromium and iron. It can be seen that after the simulated motion friction test of cartilage and stainless steel, there are two types of abrasive grains. One is the wear of the cartilage itself. The abrasive grains are round and the diameter can reach 10 microns. The abrasive grains containing iron element and chromium element obtained by peeling have a smaller diameter and long shape.

7.6.7 Abrasive Particle Analysis

The result shows the morphology of the abrasive grains observed with a microscopic system (see Figure 7-8). It can be seen that the abrasive grains are irregularly long, round, and flaky, with complex shapes and rough surfaces. The appearance is translucent. It shows the morphology of abrasive particles observed by AFM. A large number of irregular flaky, rod-shaped, circular, or filamentous abrasive particles can be seen. By scanning some of these particles, it can be seen that the shape of the abrasive particles is also more complicated. It shows the abrasive particle size distribution obtained by testing the abrasive particle size using the LS13320 laser particle size analyzer. The particle size distribution range of the abrasive particles is also examined.

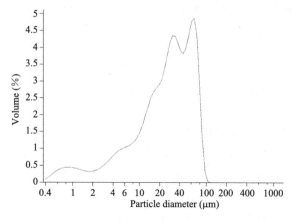

Figure 7-8   Size Distribution of Wear Particles

7.7   Analysis of Friction and Wear Mechanism of Articular Cartilage in Compound Movement Mode

7.7.1   Comparison of Test Results

Human joint motion is a composite motion of multiple motions, so the joint materials must be studied for friction and wear of joint simulation motions. In this test, the bovine articular cartilage and human articular cartilage were paired with stainless steel materials for friction and wear tests, and the friction characteristics of the material of the joints were analyzed in depth. For bovine cartilage and stainless steel, two load methods of 1000 N and 640 N were used in the simulated exercise test. The test time was divided into 20 minutes and one hour. For human cartilage and stainless steel, a load of 1000 N was used in the test for a one-hour simulated exercise test. The result shows the friction and wear performance comparison between cartilage and stainless steel cylinder under different test conditions. It can be seen that, for beef cartilage and stainless steel pairs, as the load increases from 640 N to 1000 N, after one hour of the simulated exercise test, the width and depth of the wear scars on the surface of cattle cartilage have increased greatly. Under the load, as the simulated exercise time increased from 20 minutes to one hour, the width and depth of the wear scars on the surface of cattle cartilage also increased. In the simulated exercise test of human cartilage and stainless steel pair, the load was 1000 N and the friction and wear time was one hour. Compared with bovine cartilage with the same load and time, no large damage occurred on the human cartilage surface after the test.

7.7.2　Wear Analysis

Articular cartilage is a typical two-phase material, and the liquid phase carries most of the load during exercise. Firstly, the test time is an important factor affecting cartilage wear. As the load continues to load, the loss of liquid phase carrying capacity will cause the solid-phase matrix to further increase the load, which will cause the reduced resistance to shear deformation. Therefore, with the extension of the test time, the friction properties between cartilage and stainless steel will continue to decline, and the load of the solid matrix in cartilage will continue to increase. Over time, fatigue cracking occurs on the cartilage surface material. As can be seen from ESEM observations, when the cartilage and stainless steel are simulated for 20 minutes, many strip-shaped wear marks have appeared on the contact area between the surface of the cartilage and stainless steel. Traces of cracking can be seen on the surface of the cartilage. When the area of the original cartilage on the surface of the bovine cartilage was completely worn away after one hour of movement, the calcified area of the cartilage began to appear and a large surface defect of cartilage was formed.

Secondly, the magnitude of the load also greatly affects the wear of the cartilage. In the same one-hour test, under the action of 640 N load, a large number of wear scars can be observed on the cartilage surface by ESEM. After the test, no defects of the cartilage surface layer appeared; under the action of 1000 N load, after one hour of test, a large defect appeared in the contact area between the cartilage surface and the stainless steel. Under larger loads, the load-carrying capacity of the liquid phase in cartilage decreases faster, so the accelerated fatigue damage of the solid matrix will lead to further intensification of cartilage damage and eventually cause large-scale defects in the surface structure of cartilage.

Under the load of 1000 N, after one hour of simulated kinematic friction test, the average value of the wear scar width and depth of human cartilage and bovine cartilage measured by the three-dimensional microscope system is not much different. Observing the change of cartilage surface morphology by ESEM, it can be found that large-scale defects appear on the surface of bovine cartilage, and the cartilage surface is completely worn away. However, the human cartilage surface only has large cracks, and no similar defects are found. In the existing literature

(Veeco Metrology Group, 1996), the thickness of human femur cartilage measured is greater than that of bovine femur cartilage, which plays an important role in maintaining the liquid carrying capacity of human cartilage and effectively reducing wear. In this test, although human cartilage also wears, it has thicker layers than bovine cartilage, so it can maintain good friction performance for a long time under the same load and time.

7.7.3   Comparison of Friction Between Reciprocating Motion and Compound Motion

In the reciprocating friction tests, the cartilage and the stainless steel frictional pair perform a frictional motion in a simple manner under a low load. During the friction process, the cartilage is subjected to a single load. In the composite exercise mode in this test, the movement of cartilage and stainless steel is a composite movement of internal and external rotation, flexion and extension, forward and backward displacement, and longitudinal compression force loading. The load on the cartilage is very complex. The cartilage surface is pulled and squeezed by forces in all directions. The results of composite motion wear are similar to the reciprocating friction test, but there are some differences.

In the reciprocating friction test, the cartilage and stainless steel were subjected to a reciprocating friction test under a load of 22 N for 120 minutes. As a result, it was found that a large number of abrasive particles appeared on the surface of the cartilage, uneven shapes were observed, and obvious scratches appeared. Elemental analysis found that the content of phosphorus and calcium in the wear particles on the cartilage surface was very high. It can be seen that the amorphous layer on the cartilage surface has been worn. The shape of the obtained abrasive particles is relatively regular, and the appearance of the abrasive particles is similar to spherical. Also, the number of abrasive particles of small size is large.

In the composite motion friction test, after a load of 1000 N for 20 minutes, a large number of wear particles and uneven shapes appeared on the cartilage surface. The width and depth of the wear scar on the cartilage surface were large. After one hour of simulated motion, a large area of cartilage surface was damaged. Elemental analysis showed that traces of iron were contained in the wear scars on the surface of the cartilage. After the cartilage surface was broken, chromium and iron were detected in the abrasive particles at the same time, indicating that the material transfer in stainless steel occurred, which was not found similarly in the reciprocating friction test. At the same time, compared with the reciprocating friction test, the shape of the abrasive particles produced is more irregular. There are particles which are a flake, rod, circular and filament. According to the particle size analysis, it is known that the abrasive particle size is mainly concentrated around 40, and the abrasive particle size is greater than the abrasive particles obtained in the reciprocating friction test. The wear in the friction test of the compound motion mode is abrasive wear and fatigue wear.

7.8 Summary

In this chapter, the friction pair of cartilage and stainless steel was used as the research object, and the movement of the human knee joint was simulated. The composite sports friction and wear test of cartilage sheet and stainless steel cylinder was performed on an artificial knee simulation testing machine. The main contents are as follows:

(1) After a 20-minute test under a load of 1000 N for bovine cartilage and stainless steel, there were a few wear marks on the surface of the cartilage, and the direction of the wear marks was along the contact line between the cartilage and stainless steel. Later, large damaged holes appeared on the surface of cartilage, part of the cartilage layer of the hole had been peeled off, and the subchondral bone had been exposed. After human cartilage and stainless steel were rubbed for one hour under a load of 1000 N, there were several obvious wear marks on the surface of the cartilage. There was no damage to the surface.

(2) After a one-hour test of bovine cartilage and stainless steel with a load of 640 N, there were many wear marks on the surface of the cartilage. The direction of the wear marks was along the line of contact between the cartilage and the stainless steel cylinder; as the load increased from 640 N to 1000 N, the width and depth of the wear scars on the surface of the bovine cartilage increased greatly. Under the same load, the width and depth of the wear scars on the surface of the bovine cartilage had further increased as the simulated movement time increased from 20 minutes to 1 hour.

(3) Compared with the reciprocating friction test, the composite motion friction test showed that a large number of wear particles and abrasion marks appeared on the surface of the cartilage. The transfer of metal elements could be detected in the

cartilage surface and the wear particles. This was found in the reciprocating friction test. Compared with the reciprocating friction test, the abrasive particles produced by the composite motion friction test were more irregular in shape. There were flake, rod, round, or filament abrasive particles. The size of the abrasive particle was mainly concentrated around 40 microns, which was greater than the abrasive particles obtained in the reciprocating friction test.

Chapter 8
Research on Micro Tribology and Nanomechanical Properties of Cartilage

8.1 Introduction

Gerd Binning developed the AFM on the basis of the STM in 1985. This new type of microscope, also called a scanning force microscope (SFM), can observe the surface morphology and tribological behavior of a sample at the atomic scale. The working process of AFM is as follows: The researchers bring the tip of the atomic line wide probe close to the smooth sample surface, and then use precision measurement techniques such as light deflection, light interference, capacitance, and tunnel current to detect the deformation of the flexible cantilever beam. These weak forces can be obtained after deformation. If there is a thermocouple on the tip of the needle, it can sense the temperature change and achieve the imaging of the phase boundary of the sample surface. AFM can be tested in vacuum, gas, electrochemical environment, ultra-high vacuum and solution; the sample does not have to be conductive, and can be metal, non-metal, semiconductor and polymer. After further improvement, AFM can be used to study the friction and lubrication behavior at the atomic and micron scales, and it can measure the frictional force along the sliding direction of the test surface. The stiffer probe can also be used to perform scratch and abrasion tests on the surface.

In the friction tests between solids and solids, the sample in the friction pair includes a large number of micro convex bodies on the surface, and the friction pair can contact and transfer loads through them; the scale of the AFM probe is very small, so it can be performed at the level of micro convex bodies. The study of tribology is of great significance for the further study of tribology. Articular cartilage is a typical material with a complex layered structure; during the process of friction between articular cartilage and joint material, the micro convex bodies in the sample contact and affect each other, and the interaction force will eventually cause the articular cartilage to wear. Therefore, it is necessary to use AFM to study the micro-friction and wear characteristics of articular cartilage, and use standard probes to conduct nanomechanical experiments.

8.2 Application of AFM

AFM is mainly composed of a probe, a force detection device, a position detection device, a feedback system, and an image processing and display system. The interaction between the tip of the probe and the sample surface in AFM is convenient for measuring the surface characteristics of the sample. The probe used in AFM detection is mainly composed of a cantilever and a needle tip; the shape and elastic coefficient of the probe are selected according to the needs of the test. The two commonly used operation modes are contact, non-contact and tap modes. Micro-fabricated silicon nitride probes are usually used to measure the surface morphology in contact mode; AFM in tap mode requires a rigid cantilever beam with a higher resonance frequency; AFM often uses a square prism-shaped single-crystal silicon probe manufactured by etching. In the test, AFM can simulate the contact of micro convex bodies between materials and can attach silicon balls and the like to the probe head for measurement as the needle tip (Veeco Metrology Group, 1999).

During the measurement, the test sample is mounted on a piezoelectric ceramic tube scanner (PZT). PZT can realize small displacement, so it can control the accurate scanning of the sample in the space x direction and y direction, and move the sample in the vertical z direction. The laser beam generated by the laser passes through the prism; after it is guided to the back of the cantilever end, the beam is reflected on the back of the cantilever, and then guided by a beam splitter to a four-quadrant photodetector (PSPD). The AFM measurement system uses the differential signals from the upper and lower photodetectors to obtain the vertical deflection of the cantilever. When the probe scans the sample, the vertical change of the sample surface causes the probe to deviate vertically, and then the direction of the reflected laser light is changed accordingly. Finally, it can change the intensity difference between the upper and lower photodetectors. When measuring the surface topography, the normal force exerted on the probe is kept constant. Also, the height of the PZT must be continuously adjusted by the feedback circuit during the measurement; the height adjustment makes the deflection of the cantilever during the scanning process unchanged, and the height of the PZT adjustment reflects the fluctuation of the surface of the sample.

In the working mode of measuring friction force, the photodetector in the left and right quadrants is used to detect the deflection of the laser during the probe sliding measurement on the sample surface. During the test, the friction between the sample and the probe caused the cantilever to distort. After the laser beam was reflected from the torsional plane on the back of the cantilever, it was received by the photodetectors in the left and right quadrants. The resulting intensity difference was the friction voltage signal. The difference in the torsion angle changes the strength difference, which can be converted into the magnitude of the friction force. The slope of the friction force and the normal force change can be used to obtain the friction factor.

8.3　Test Method

8.3.1　Sample Preparation and Test Equipment

The test instruments are Nanoscope-III AFM (Shanghai Jiao Tong University Analytical Testing Center, American DI Company). Samples of human cartilage pins, bovine cartilage pins and PVA hydrogel pins with a diameter of 12 mm were obtained after processing the samples; the thickness of the samples was about 3 mm. The PVA hydrogel was chemically crosslinked. In the test, 15% PVA was used to dissolve in the DMSO aqueous solution, and the solution was obtained after freezing and thawing. The probes used in the tests were also observed using SEM. A silicon nitride probe was used in the micro friction test. Its normal elastic coefficient was 0.06 N/m, the length was 200 microns, and the diameter of the probe tip was about 40 nm. In order to achieve accelerated wear during the test, a silicon probe with a large elastic coefficient was used in the micro-wear test; the probe had a normal elastic coefficient of 2.5 N/m, a length of 125 microns, and a needle tip diameter of 10 nm. In the test, the feedback voltage signal was taken to indicate the magnitude of the friction force. The same sample was measured at three positions and then averaged.

8.3.2   Probe Modification

In the test, it is necessary to simulate the contact between the micro convex bodies, which is one of the implementation methods of the cartilage micro friction test; therefore, before the test, the researchers affixed the glass microspheres to the probe head as the needle tip to perform the friction test with the sample. Glass microspheres are 12 borosilicate glass spheres produced by the Shanghai Institute of Metrology and Testing Technology. In the institute, a micromanipulator is used to paste glass microspheres. The glue is special glass glue (PATTEX series). The installation of glass microspheres requires multiple steps (Veeco Metrology Group, 1996). The probes with the glass microspheres are also observed with SEM (see Figure 8-1).

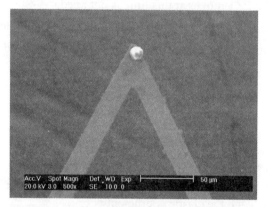

Figure 8-1   Probes Attached Glass Microsphere

The specific process is as follows:

(1) Install two thin metal wires on the micromanipulator, and place the AFM probe on the lower part of the wire on the glass slide;

(2) Put a small amount of glue on the surface of the slide, and use the end of the first metal wire to dip a small amount of glue;

(3) Apply the glue dipped at the end of the metal wire to the part of the cantilever where the glass microspheres need to be pasted;

(4) Use the second metal wire to place the glass microspheres on the cantilever to apply the glue, and wait until it is dry.

8.3.3   Probe Calibration

After the glass microspheres are attached to the probe, the elastic coefficient will change, so the elastic coefficient needs to be recalibrated. In this test, the calibration operation was performed according to the method proposed by Ruan & Bhushan (1994). Take the standard cantilever sample for testing during calibration. The standard cantilever sample is fixedly mounted on the fixed end of the PZT, and one side is in contact with the cantilever being tested. Specific steps are as follows:

(1) Use a probe to be calibrated to measure a high-hardness specimen (such as a gemstone), and make sure that the distance that PZT moves (measured from the contact point between the probe and the specimen) is equal to the deflection distance of the cantilever.

(2) Measure the standard cantilever sample. Because the standard cantilever test is an elastic body, in order to keep the cantilever deflection consistent level, the distance at which the PZT moves at this time is obtained.

(3) The difference between the two moving distances is related to the deflection of the standard sample. The elastic coefficient of the measured cantilever can be calculated as follows:

$$(Z_t' - Z_t)k_s = Z_t k_c.$$

Get the coefficient of elasticity:

$$k_c = k_s(Z_t' - Z_t)/Z_t.$$

Among them, the distance that PZT moves is Z_t, the distance that PZT moves the second time is Z_t', and the elastic coefficient is k_s.

The standard cantilever sample used for calibration in this test has a coefficient of elasticity of 0.083 N/m, a length of 383 microns, a width of 31 microns, a thickness of 2.38 microns, a resonance frequency of 21.23 kHz, a density of 2330 kg/m^3, and Young's modulus: 1.52×10^{11} N/m^3. The elastic coefficient of the modified probe is calculated according to the above formula to be 0.092 N/m. After the conversion, it can be known that the 1 V signal represents approximately 4.5816 nN load when the load is applied.

8.4 Micro Friction Test of Cartilage

In the experiment, probes with glass microspheres were used for the experiments. The samples included bovine cartilage, human cartilage and PVA hydrogel artificial cartilage. The effects of load and speed on friction were studied in the test. AFM uses the liquid environment observation mode, and the liquid environment at this time is physiological saline. The test scanning area is a 25-micron square, and the friction voltage signal value is the average of the voltages for the forward and return journeys. In the friction and load test, the scanning length is 25 microns, the speed is constant at 10 microns per second, and the pressure is 0–18 volts. In the friction and speed test, the scanning length was 25 microns, the speeds were 5, 25, 50, 100, 150, 200, 250, 300, 350 and 400 microns per second and the load voltage was 12 volts. Friction voltage is the average of the difference between the forward and return voltages.

8.4.1　Effect of Load on Friction

After the experiment, the relationship of the friction between the different samples and the probe with the load was obtained (see Figure 8-2). With the increase of the load, the friction between the different samples and the probe showed an upward trend. When the load is 0 volts, the probe does not have any force on the cartilage surface, but the friction of the probe on the surface will still produce friction. This indicates the existence of the adhesion between the sample and the probe. Such adhesive force can produce a friction force of about 10 volts, which is the result of van der Waals force.

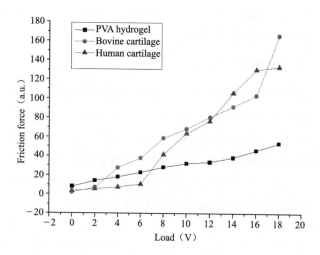

Figure 8-2　Variation of Friction Forces with Loads

The slope of the test curve represents the friction coefficient of different materials. The results show that when the load increases, the micro friction coefficient of natural cartilage has been increasing, and the friction coefficient of artificial cartilage has not changed much. It can be seen that natural cartilage in micro friction is not applicable to the conclusion that the coefficient of friction in Amontons formula has nothing to do with contact area and load. Derjaguin had modified the Amontons formula as follows:

$$F = F_0 + \mu L.$$

The left side of the formula represents the total load that the sample is subjected to, the first term on the right side of the formula is the adhesion force under zero load, and the second term on the right side is the product of the externally applied load and the friction coefficient. According to the revised formula, in this test, when the load changes, the adhesion force generated by the contact between the probe or cartilage and artificial cartilage will change with the test conditions, which will cause friction coefficient change. Under the lower load at the beginning of the test, the friction between natural cartilage and artificial cartilage is very close, but as the load increases, the friction coefficient of natural cartilage changes greatly, but the friction coefficient of artificial cartilage changes little. This may be related to the lack of boundary lubricants on the surface of the PVA hydrogel and thus the lower adhesion. Under the same load conditions, it can be found from the results that the frictional force between bovine cartilage or human cartilage and the probe varies in the same range, and the difference is not obvious.

8.4.2   Effect of Speed on Friction

As a result, the relationship between the friction between different samples and the probe as a function of scanning speed is obtained (see Figure 8-3). It is found that the sliding speed has a significant effect on the friction force, which is mainly manifested in different performances at different speed changing stages. When the speed increases in the range of 0–100, the friction between the sample and the probe gradually increases. When the speed increases in the range of 100–250, the friction force obtained in the test can be maintained in a certain range. When the speed increases in the range of 250–400, the friction between the sample and the probe begins to gradually increase; at this time, the natural cartilage growth is not obvious, and the growth of the PVA hydrogel is more obvious. When the sample and the probe are rubbed at a lower speed, the micro convex bodies on the sample surface will elastically deform after contact with the probe; the micro convex bodies that undergo elastic deformation make the probe easier to scratch the surface of the sample. As the scanning speed increases, the micro convex body will not be deformed in time. Therefore, as the speed increases, the friction force will increase. At this time, the ratchet effect of micro friction will work. When the micro convex body can no longer respond to the sliding of the probe, the friction force will reach a nearly constant state. When the scanning speed exceeds 250, part of the micro convex on the sample surface may have been scratched. At this time, the furrow effect works; the surface of the sample will gather materials, making the sample surface more uneven, and the friction will be rising. It can be found in the results that the friction between natural cartilage and PVA hydrogel artificial cartilage test is quite different. From the results of the compression mechanics test, it can be seen that the compression modulus of natural cartilage is greater than that of PVA hydrogel. Therefore, during the contact process of the probe with natural cartilage and PVA hydrogel, the deformation of PVA hydrogel is greater than that of natural cartilage. It will reduce the twist of the probe and thus reduce the friction.

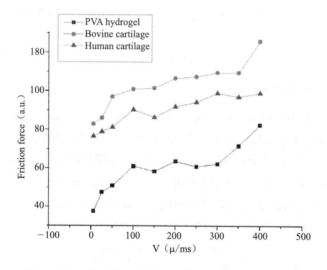

Figure 8-3   Variation of Friction Forces with Scan Speed

8.5   Micro-Wear Test of Cartilage

In the micro-wear test, the AFM probe was used to study the micro-wear properties of bovine cartilage and PVA hydrogel, and the wear morphology of the samples was also observed. In order to accelerate the wear, a probe with a large elastic coefficient is used, and a silicon probe with an elastic coefficient of 2.5 N/m is used for the wear test. When a load is applied, the 1 V signal represents a load of 124.5 nN. Before the wear test, the surface of each sample is observed to establish and determine the benchmark for the depth of wear, and at the same time to observe the presence of contaminants on the surface to prevent the wear test from being affected. Next, wear tests are performed at selected locations. The scanning range of the probe is a square area of 10 micrometers, and the wear range of the probe is 5 micrometers at the center. The wear process is as follows. First, the probe slides along the lateral direction for 5 micrometers and then moves a small step along the transverse direction. The probe slides backward for 5 micrometers, and finally reaches the set wear time. A square worn surface was found. According to the test requirements, the time and load of wear are specified. The amount of wear during the wear process is very small. In order to measure the change in the amount of wear, a method of measuring the depth of wear is used for research. In the test of the influence of friction time on wear, a load of 4 V was used, and in the test of the influence of load on wear, the friction time was 10 minutes. AFM's new probe tip is sharp and prone to wear, which can cause errors in the wear test. Before the test, the probe tip is blunt, and then the test is performed.

8.5.1 Effect of Friction Time on Wear

As a result, the relationship between the wear scar depth of bovine cartilage and PVA hydrogel as a function of friction time was obtained (see Figure 8-4). In addition, surface observations of bovine cartilage and PVA hydrogel at different times were also obtained. When rubbed for 10 minutes, there are slight wear marks on the surface of bovine cartilage and PVA hydrogel, and the accumulation of material in the center of the surface of bovine cartilage is caused by the transfer of materials during the abrasion process. When rubbed for 20 minutes, the surface of bovine cartilage has obvious wear marks, and the PVA hydrogel also has obvious wear marks. The wear of the bovine cartilage surface appears as the appearance of pits, and the wear of PVA hydrogel appears as the expansion of the original holes on the surface. After the same wear time, the wear depth of bovine cartilage is greater than that of PVA hydrogel.

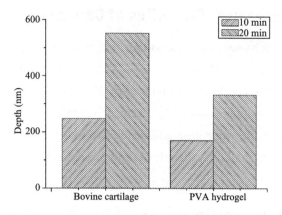

Figure 8-4   Depth of Grinding Crack with Sliding Time

8.5.2   Effect of Load on Wear

As a result, the change of wear scar depth of bovine cartilage and PVA hydrogel with load was obtained (see Figure 8-5). With the increase of the load, the wear depth increases, and it can be seen that the wear of bovine cartilage and PVA hydrogel has different trends with the change of load. When the load is low, the amount of wear of bovine cartilage is low. When the load is increased to 4 V, the amount of wear of bovine cartilage rises quickly. Because the surface of bovine cartilage has an amorphous layer rich in boundary lubricants when the load is large, the amorphous layer is quickly destroyed, and pits and material accumulation have already appeared, which will cause a rapid rise in wear. The surface material of PVA hydrogel is single and has no layered structure, so the wear changes relatively smoothly with the load.

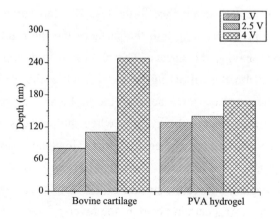

Figure 8-5   Depth of Grinding Crack with Different Loads

8.6 Nanomechanical Properties of Cartilage

In the nanomechanical test, a nano-indentation test is performed on the surface of the sample using an AFM tapered probe. The tapered probe is a silicon nitride probe with an elastic coefficient of 0.06 N/m. For infinitely rigid specimens, the deformation of the probe is equal to the distance the material moves at the probe. For soft material testing, the probe head will be pressed into the sample, and the depth of the push will cause a small piezoelectric platform to deform:

$$d = z - \delta.$$

As a result, the force curve is flatter and the slope is smaller. With the applied force F and elastic coefficient k, according to Hooke's law, the equation is:

$$F = kd = k(z - \delta).$$

Sneddon extended the model proposed by Hertz to obtain a model for the indentation of flat specimens by cones. The model formula is as follows:

$$F = (2/\pi)[E/(1 - v^2)]\delta^2\tan(\alpha).$$

According to the Hertz formula, the obtained force curve is fitted, and the above two formulas are obtained:

$$z - z_0 = d - d_0 + \sqrt{\frac{k(d - d_0)}{(2/\pi)[E/(1 - v^2)]\tan(\alpha)}}.$$

Without deformation, the Poisson ratio is 0.5, and the elastic coefficient of the probe is 8 mN/m. As a result, the calculation force curve can be obtained.

The force curve can be obtained in the test. The left curve in the result is the force curve of the probe pressing into the surface, and the right curve is the force curve of the probe leaving the surface. The process of pressing the probe into the sample is divided into the following processes: when the probe approaches the sample surface, the attractive force between the probe and the surface atoms of the sample pulls the probe toward the sample; when the probe is in contact with the sample surface, the load begins to be applied. As the load increases, the probe deflects more, and the contact force increases sharply. After the load is applied to a certain extent, the probe begins to leave the surface of the sample. The needle will deflect in the opposite direction. At a certain position, the reverse force and the adhesive force are equal. After that, the probe bounces off the sample surface.

Take multiple points on the surface of each sample to perform mechanical tests to obtain the elastic modulus of different samples. After calculation, the elastic modulus of bovine joint cartilage is 598 ± 102 kPa, and the elastic modulus of human joint cartilage is 605 ± 263 kPa. The hydrogel elastic modulus is 634 ± 155 kPa. It can be seen that the nanomechanical modulus of cartilage and artificial cartilage is lower than the test results in the macro compression test. The elastic modulus of PVA hydrogel is greater than that of bovine cartilage and human cartilage. The elastic modulus of human cartilage is different from that of bovine cartilage. In the nanomechanical test, the probe is pressed into an amorphous layer on the cartilage surface. From the test results, it can be found that the amorphous layer is more likely to deform than the surface of the PVA hydrogel.

8.7　Micro Friction and Macro Friction Wear

In macroscopic tribology research on cartilage and artificial cartilage, it is generally believed that the increase of cartilage friction coefficient is related to the change of the two-phase properties of cartilage. During the process of cartilage loading, the continuous loss of the liquid phase will cause the liquid phase to withstand the load reduction. After the solid phase bearing load increases, the contact between the solid phase and the solid phase will cause the friction coefficient to increase. However, the influence of the surface micro convex contact in friction cannot be reflected, and the micro friction wear test is a good research approach.

In the study of micro friction, both friction pairs are in the micro-contact state: first, the contact state of micro convex bodies can be simulated; second, the mechanism of friction force generation in macro friction can be explained. At the same time, micro friction has the characteristics of small scale and low load. These characteristics can remove the effects of two-phase performance and hydrodynamic lubrication in cartilage friction, and only consider the influence of surface contact and the surface boundary lubrication layer. There are three main friction mechanisms in micro friction, including adhesion mechanism, ratchet mechanism and furrow mechanism. Due to the presence of an amorphous layer on the surface of natural cartilage in micro friction, the load makes the probe and the boundary lubrication component in the amorphous layer interact more easily; physical or chemical adhesion occurs between them, which will cause friction. At the same time, the ratchet and furrow effect in the contact between the probe and the micro convex body on the sample surface will also generate friction. When the probe is drawn across the surface of the sample, the micro convex body will not be deformed or slightly deformed as the probe passes. At this time, the micro friction ratchet effect works. When the micro friction time is long or the load is large, the micro convex body on the test surface will be deformed, and the micro convex body may be partially scratched. Also, the furrow effect works.

The microwear test can simulate the wear conditions that occur during the contact of the micro convex body, which is equivalent to the situation immediately after the wear in the macro friction test. From the results of the micro-wear test, it can be seen that the forms of wear on the surface of bovine cartilage and PVA hydrogel are different; the wear of bovine cartilage appears like the appearance of pits, and also includes the accumulation of a large amount of surface material around. Abrasion is manifested by the expansion of surface holes. With the increase of pits on the surface of bovine cartilage and the continuous accumulation of material, particles of material accumulation will appear on the worn surface of bovine cartilage, which has been found in macroscopic friction tests. At the same time, the pits on the surface of bovine cartilage are further deepened, and as a result, the cartilage surface is damaged. The expansion of pores on the surface of PVA hydrogel will cause surface cracking, the surface material is easy to peel off from the surface, and it will cause the adhesion phenomenon that occurs in the macro friction test.

8.8 Summary

The AFM was used to study the micro friction properties of cartilage and PVA hydrogel artificial cartilage. In the research, a probe modification method was used for the test. Before the test, a micromanipulator was used, the glass microspheres were pasted on the needle part of the silicon nitride probe, and then the friction test was performed using the tip as a tip and the sample.

In the micro friction test, as the load rises, the friction between different samples and the probe shows an upward trend. When the load is increased, the microscopic friction coefficient of natural cartilage has been increasing, and the friction coefficient of artificial cartilage has not changed much.

The sliding speed has a significant effect on the friction force. When the speed increases in the range of 0 to 100 microns per second, the friction between the sample and the probe gradually increases. When the speed increases in the range of 100 to

250 microns per second, the friction obtained in the test can be maintained within a certain range. When the speed increases in the range of 250 to 400 microns per second, the friction between the sample and the probe begins to gradually increase. At this time, the growth of natural cartilage is not obvious, and the growth of PVA hydrogel is more obvious. When the sample and the probe are rubbed at a lower speed, the micro convex bodies on the sample surface will elastically deform after contact with the probe. The elastically deformed micro convex bodies make the probe easier to scratch the surface of the sample. As the scanning speed increases, the micro convex body will not be deformed in time, and as the speed increases, the friction force will increase. At this time, the ratchet effect of micro friction will work. When the micro convex body can no longer respond to the sliding of the probe, the friction force will reach a nearly constant state. When the scanning speed is very large, the micro convex body on the sample surface may have been scratched. At this time, the furrow effect works, the material on the sample surface gathers, making the sample surface more uneven, and the friction force rises at the same time.

The AFM was used to study the micro-wear properties of bovine cartilage and PVA hydrogel. The wear scar depth of bovine cartilage and PVA hydrogel increased with increasing friction time. With the increase of the load, the wear depth increases, and the wear of bovine cartilage and PVA hydrogel has different trends with the change of load. When the load is low, the wear amount of bovine cartilage is low. When the load is increased to 4 V, the bovine cartilage is worn. The amount of wear rises quickly. The wear of bovine cartilage is manifested by the appearance of pits and the accumulation of a large number of surrounding materials, and the wear of PVA hydrogel is represented by the expansion of surface holes. After the abrasion of bovine cartilage is aggravated, particles formed after the material is peeled off will accumulate on the surface, and the surface pits will further aggravate the cartilage surface damage. The expansion of pores on the surface of the PVA hydrogel will cause surface cracking, and the surface material will be easily peeled from the surface, which will cause the adhesion phenomenon in the macro friction test.

In the nanomechanical test, an AFM is used to perform a nano-micro indentation test on the surface of the sample. The nanomechanical elastic modulus of cartilage and artificial cartilage is lower than the test results in the macro compression test. The elastic modulus of PVA hydrogel is greater than that of bovine cartilage and human cartilage.

References

[1] A. A. Spirt, A. F. Mak & R. P. Wassell. Nonlinear Viscoelastic Properties of Articular Cartilage in Shear [J]. *Journal of Orthopaedic Research*, 1989, *7* (1): 43-49.

[2] A. Chiba, S. Sakakura, K. Kobayashi & K. Kusayanagi. Dissolution Amounts of Nickel, Chromium and Iron from Sus 304, 316 and 444 Stainless Steels in Sodium Chloride Solutions [J]. *Journal of Materials Science*, 1997, *32* (8): 1995-2000.

[3] A. F. Mak, W. M. Lai & V. C. Mow. Biphasic Indentation of Articular Cartilage-I. Theoretical Analysis [J]. *Journal of Biomechanics*, 1987, *20* (7): 703-714.

[4] A. J. Smith. *A Study of the Forces on the Body in Athletic Activities, with Particular Reference to Jumping* [M]. Leeds: University of Leeds, 1972.

[5] A. M. Trunfio-Sfarghiu, Y. Berthier, M. H. Meurisse & J. P. Rieu. Multiscale Analysis of the Tribological Role of the Molecular Assemblies of Synovial Fluid: Case of a Healthy Joint and Implants [J]. *Tribology International*, 2007, *40* (10-12 SPEC. ISS.): 1500-1515.

[6] A. N. Suciu, T. Iwatsubo, M. Matsuda & T. Nishino. Wear Characteristics of a Novel Bearing System for Artificial Knee Joint (Micro-Pocket-Covered Femoral Component and Tibial Poro-Elastic-Hydrated Cartilage) [J]. *JSME International Journal, Series C: Mechanical Systems, Machine Elements and Manufacturing*, 2004, *47* (1): 209-217.

[7] A. Unsworth. Recent Developments in the Tribology of Artificial Joints [J]. *Tribology International*, 1995, *28* (7): 485-495.

[8] A. Unsworth, D. Dowson & V. Wright. Some New Evidence on Human Joint Lubrication [J]. *Annals of the Rheumatic Diseases*, 1975, *34* (4): 277-285.

[9] A. Wang, A. Essner, C. Stark & J. H. Dumbleton. A Biaxial Line-Contact Wear Machine for the Evaluation of Implant Bearing Materials for Total Knee Joint Replacement [J]. *Wear*, 1999, *225-229* (2): 701-707.

[10] A. W. Neumann, D. R. Absolom, D. W. Francis & C. J. V. Oss. Conversion Tables of Contact Angles to Surface Tensions [J]. *Separation and Purification Methods*, 1980, *9* (1): 69-163.

[11] B. A. Hills. Boundary Lubrication *in Vivo* [J]. *Proceedings of the Institution of Mechanical Engineers, Part H: Journal of Engineering in Medicine*, 2000, *214* (1): 83-94.

[12] B. A. Hills. Oligolamellar Lubrication of Joints by Surface Active Phospholipid [J]. *Journal of Rheumatology*, 1989, *16* (1): 82-91.

[13] B. A. Hills. Remarkable Anti-Wear Properties of Joint Surfactant [J]. *Annals of Biomedical Engineering*, 1995, *23* (2): 112-115.

[14] B. A. Hills & B. D. Buttler. Surfactants Identified in Synovial Fluid and Their Ability to Act as Boundary Lubricants [J]. *Annals of the Rheumatic Diseases*, 1984, *43* (4): 641-648.

[15] B. Wang, S. Mukataka, E. Kokufuta & M. Kodama. The Influence of Polymer Concentration on the Radiation-Chemical Yield of Intermolecular Crosslinking of Poly (Vinyl Alcohol) by Gamma-Rays in Deoxygenated Aqueous Solution [J]. *Radiation Physics and Chemistry*, 2000, *59* (1): 91-95.

[16] C. C. B. Wang, J. M. Deng, G. A. Ateshian & C. T. Hung. An Automated Approach for Direct Measurement of Two-Dimensional Strain Distributions within Articular Cartilage Under Unconfined Compression [J]. *Journal of Biomechanical Engineering*, 2002, *124* (5): 557-567.

[17] C. G. Armstrong & V. C. Mow. Variations in the Intrinsic Mechanical Properties of Human Articular Cartilage with Age, Degeneration, and Water Content [J]. *Journal of Bone and Joint Surgery—Series A*, 1982, *64* (1): 88-94.

[18] C. J. V. Oss & C. F. Gillman. Phagocytosis as a Surface Phenomenon. Contact Angles and Phagocytosis of Non-Opsonized Bacteria [J]. *RES Journal of the Reticuloendothelial Society*, 1972, *12* (3): 283-292.

[19] C. R. Orford & D. L. Gardner. Ultrastructural Histochemistry of the Surface Lamina of Normal Articular Cartilage [J]. *Histochemical Journal*, 1985, *17* (2): 223-233.

[20] C. W. McCutchen. The Frictional Properties of Animal Joints [J]. *Wear*, 1962, *5*

(1): 1-17.

[21] D. Dowson. *Are Our Joint Replacement Materials Adequate? Proceedings of International Conference on the Changing Role of Engineering in Orthopaedics* [M]. Unpublished: 1989.

[22] D. Dowson. *Bio-Tribology of Natural and Replacement Synovial Joints* [M]. Berlin: Springer Verlag, 1990.

[23] D. Dowson. *History of Tribology* [M]. Hoboken: Wiley, 1998.

[24] D. Dowson & V. Wright. *The Reology of Lubricants* [M]. Leeds: Institute of Petroleum of University of Leeds, 1973.

[25] D. Dowson & V. Wright. *An Introduction to the Bio-Mechanics of Joints and Joint Replacement* [M]. Hoboken: Wiley-Blackwell, 1981.

[26] D. Eyrich, F. Brandl, B. Appel, H. Wiese, G. Maier, M. Wenzel, R. Staudenmaier, A. Goepferich & T. Blunk. Long-Term Stable Fibrin Gels for Cartilage Engineering [J]. *Biomaterials*, 2007, *28* (1): 55-65.

[27] D. H. Hoch, A. J. Grodzinsky & T. J. Koob. Early Changes in Material Properties of Rabbit Articular Cartilage After Meniscectomy [J]. *Journal of Orthopaedic Research*, 1983, *1* (1): 4-12.

[28] D. J. DiAngelo & I. A. Harrington. *Design of a Dynamic Multi-Purpose Joint Simulato* [M]. New York: American Society of Mechanical Engineers, 1992.

[29] D. L. Gardner, P. O'Connor, K. Oates. Low Temperature Scanning Electron Microscopy of Dog and Guinea-Pig Hyaline Articular Cartilage [J]. *Journal of Anatomy*, 1981, *132* (2): 267-282.

[30] D. Xiong & S. Ge. Friction and Wear Properties of Uhmwpe/Al2o3 Ceramic Under Different Lubricating Conditions [J]. *Wear*, 2001, *250* (1): 242-245.

[31] E. P. J. Watters, P. L. Spedding, J. Grimshaw, J. M. Duffy & R.L. Spedding. Wear of Artificial Hip Joint Material [J]. *Chemical Engineering Journal*, 2005, *112* (1-3): 137-144.

[32] E. S. Grood & W. J. Suntay. A Joint Coordinate System for the Clinical Description of Three-Dimensional Motions: Application to the Knee [J]. *Journal of Biomechanical Engineering*, 1983, *105* (2): 136-144.

[33] E. Wachtel, A. Maroudas & R. Schneiderman. Age-Related Changes in Collagen Packing of Human Articular Cartilage [J]. *Biochimica et Biophysica Acta-General Subjects*, 1995, *1243* (2): 239-243.

[34] F. Eckstein, B. Lemberger, T. Stammberger, K. H. Englmeier & M. Reiser.

Patellar Cartilage Deformation *in Vivo* After Static Versus Dynamic Loading [J]. *Journal of Biomechanics*, 2000, *33* (7): 819-825.

[35] F. Eckstein, M. Reiser, K. H. Englmeier & R. Putz. *In Vivo* Morphometry and Functional Analysis of Human Articular Cartilage with Quantitative Magnetic Resonance Imaging—from Image to Data, from Data to Theory [J]. *Anatomy and Embryology*, 2001, *203* (3): 147-173.

[36] F. N. Ghadially. *Fine Structure of Synovial Joints: A Text and Atlas of the Ultrastructure of Normal and Pathological Articular Tissues* [M]. Oxford: Butterworth-Heinemann, 1983.

[37] G. A. Ateshian & C. T. Hung. The Natural Synovial Joint: Properties of Cartilage [J]. *Proceedings of the Institution of Mechanical Engineers, Part J: Journal of Engineering Tribology*, 2006, *220* (8): 657-670.

[38] G. E. Kempson, C. J. Spivey, S. A. V. Swanson & M. A. R. Freeman. Patterns of Cartilage Stiffness on Normal and Degenerate Human Femoral Heads [J]. *Journal of Biomechanics*, 1971, *4* (6): 597-609, IN525-IN526.

[39] G. E. Kempson, M. A. R. Freeman & S. A. V. Swanson. The Determination of a Creep Modulus for Articular Cartilage from Indentation Tests on the Human Femoral Head [J]. *Journal of Biomechanics*, 1971, *4* (4): 239-250.

[40] G. P. Dempsey & S. Bullivant. A Copper Block Method for Freezing Non-Cryoprotected Tissue to Produce Ice Crystal Free Regions for Electron Microscopy. I. Evaluation Using Freeze Substitution [J]. *Journal of Microscopy*, 1976, *106* (3): 251-260.

[41] G. W. Blunn, A. B. Joshi, R. J. Minns, L. Lidgren, P. Lilley, L. Ryd, E. Engelbrecht & P. S. Walker. Wear in Retrieved Condylar Knee Arthroplasties: A Comparison of Wear in Different Designs of 280 Retrieved Condylar Knee Prostheses [J]. *Journal of Arthroplasty*, 1997, *12* (3): 281-290.

[42] G. Wu, C. Zhao, C. Wang & W. Zhang. The Effect of Preparation Methods on Tribological Properties of Pva-H/Ha Composites [J]. *Iranian Polymer Journal (English Edition)*, 2008, *17* (11): 811-819.

[43] H. Bodugoz-Senturk, C. E. Macias, J. H. Kung & O. K. Muratoglu. Poly (Vinyl Alcohol)-Acrylamide Hydrogels as Load-Bearing Cartilage Substitute [J]. *Biomaterials*, 2009, *30* (4): 589-596.

[44] H. Forster & J. Fisher. The Influence of Continuous Sliding and Subsequent Surface Wear on the Friction of Articular Cartilage [J]. *Proceedings of the*

Institution of Mechanical Engineers, Part H: Journal of Engineering in Medicine, 1999, *213* (4): 329-345.

[45] H. Higaki, T. Murakami, Y. Nakanishi, H. Miura, T. Mawatari & Y. Inamoto. The Lubricating Ability of Biomembrane Models with Dipalmitoyl Phosphatidylcholine and Gamma-Globulin [J]. *Proceedings of the Institution of Mechanical Engineers, Part H: Journal of Engineering in Medicine*, 1998, *212* (5): 337-346.

[46] H. J. Agins, N. W. Alcock, M. Bansal, E. A. Salvati, P. D. Wilson Jr., P. M. Pellicci & P. G. Bullough. Metallic Wear in Failed Titanium-Alloy Total Hip Replacements: A Histological and Quantitative Analysis [J]. *Journal of Bone and Joint Surgery—Series A*, 1988, *70* (3): 347-356.

[47] H. J. Fruh & G. Willmann. Tribological Investigations of the Wear Couple Alumina-Cfrp for Total Hip Replacement [J]. *Biomaterials*, 1998, *19* (13): 1145-1150.

[48] H. Liang, B. Shi, A. Fairchild & T. Cale. Applications of Plasma Coatings in Artificial Joints: An Overview [J]. *Vacuum*, 2004, *73* (3-4): 317-326.

[49] H. Nakae, R. Inui, Y. Hirata & H. Saito. Effects of Surface Roughness on Wettability [J]. *Acta Materialia*, 1998, *46* (7): 2313-2318.

[50] H. N. Shih, L. Y. Shih, Y. C. Wong & R. W. W. Hsu. Long-Term Changes of the Nonresurfaced Patella After Total Knee Arthroplasty [J]. *Journal of Bone and Joint Surgery—Series A*, 2004, *86* (5): 935-939.

[51] H. Trieu & S. Qutubuddin. Poly (Vinyl Alcohol) Hydrogels: 2. Effects of Processing Parameters on Structure and Properties [J]. *Polymer*, 1995, *36* (13): 2531-2539.

[52] I. Langmuir & V. J. Schaefer. The Effect of Dissolved Salts on Insoluble Monolayers [J]. *Journal of the American Chemical Society*, 1937, *59* (11): 2400-2414.

[53] T. Inoue. Gelled Vinyl Alcohol Polymers and Articles Therefrom [P]. In U. Patent (Ed.) *United States Patent and Trademark Office Granted Patent.* Washington: United States Patent and Trademark Office, 1975.

[54] ISO. *Implants for Surgery-Wear of Total Knee-Joint Prostheses—Part 1: Loading and Displacement Parameters for Wear-Testing Machines with Load Control and Corresponding Environmental Conditions for Test* [S]. Geneva: International Organization for Standardization, 2002.

[55] ISO. *Implants for Surgery-Wear of Total Knee-Joint Prostheses—Part 3: Loading and Displacement Parameters for Wear-Testing Machines with Displacement Control and Corresponding Environmental Conditions for Test* [S]. Geneva: International Organization for Standardization, 2004.

[56] ISO. *Implants for Surgery-Wear of Total Knee-Hip Joint Prostheses—Part 2: Methods of Measurement* [S]. Geneva: International Organization for Standardization, 2000.

[57] J. A. Ruan & B. Bhushan. Atomic-Scale Friction Measurements Using Friction Force Microscopy: Part I—General Principles and New Measurement Techniques [J]. *Journal of Tribology*, 1994, *116* (2): 378-388.

[58] J. B. Stiehl, R. D. Komistek, D. A. Dennis & P. A. Keblish. Kinematics of the Patellofemoral Joint in Total Knee Arthroplasty [J]. *Journal of Arthroplasty*, 2001, *16* (6): 706-714.

[59] J. Bo. Study on Pva Hydrogel Crosslinked by Epichlorohydrin [J]. *Journal of Applied Polymer Science*, 1992, *46* (5): 783-786.

[60] J. C. Waterton, S. Solloway, J. E. Foster, M. C. Keen, S. Gandy, B. J. Middleton, R. A. Maciewicz, I. Watt, P. A. Dieppe & C. J. Taylor. Diurnal Variation in the Femoral Articular Cartilage of the Knee in Young Adult Humans [J]. *Magnetic Resonance in Medicine*, 2000, *43* (1): 126-132.

[61] J. Charnley. The Lubrication of Animal Joints in Relation to Surgical Reconstruction by Arthroplasty [J]. *Annals of the Rheumatic Diseases*, 1960, *19* (1): 10-19.

[62] J. Chappuis, I. A. Sherman & A. W. Neumann. Surface Tension of Animal Cartilage as It Relates to Friction in Joints [J]. *Annals of Biomedical Engineering*, 1983, *11* (5): 435-449.

[63] J. D. Desjardins, P. S. Walker, H. Haider & J. Perry. The Use of a Force-Controlled Dynamic Knee Simulator to Quantify the Mechanical Performance of Total Knee Replacement Designs During Functional Activity [J]. *Journal of Biomechanics*, 2000, *33* (10): 1231-1242.

[64] J. F. Hersh, B. M. Hillberry & D. B. Kettelkamp. Laboratory Knee Simulation Testing, Preliminary Results on Three Prostheses [J]. *Transaction Orthopaedic Research Society*, 1981 (6): 211.

[65] J. Insall, W. N. Scott & C. S. Ranawat. The Total Condylar Knee Prosthesis: A Report of Two Hundred and Twenty Cases [J]. *Journal of Bone and Joint*

Surgery—Series A, 1979, *61* (2): 173-180.

[66] J. G. Peyron & E. A. Balazs. Preliminary Clinical Assessment of Na-Hyaluronate Injection into Human Arthritic Joints [J]. *Pathologie Biologie*, 1974, *22* (8): 731-736.

[67] J. H. Dumbleton. *Tribology of Natural and Artificial Joints* [M]. Amsterdam: Elsevier Scientific Publishing Company, 1981.

[68] J. J. Elias, M. Kumagai, I. Mitchell, Y. Mizuno, S. M. Mattessich, J. D. Webb & E. Y. Chao. *In Vitro* Kinematic Patterns Are Similar for a Fixed Platform and a Mobile Bearing Prosthesis [J]. *Journal of Arthroplasty*, 2002, *17* (4): 467-474.

[69] J. I. Oate, M. Comin, I. Braceras, A. Garcia, J. L. Viviente, M. Brizuela, N. Garagorri, J. L. Peris & J. I. Alava. Wear Reduction Effect on Ultra-High-Molecular-Weight Polyethylene by Application of Hard Coatings and Ion Implanation on Cobalt Chromium Ally, as Measured in a Knee Wear Simulation Machine [J]. *Surface and Coatings Technology*, 2001 (142-144): 1056-1062.

[70] J. Katta, S. S. Pawaskar, Z. M. Jin, E. Ingham & J. Fisher. Effect of Load Variation on the Friction Properties of Articular Cartilage [J]. *Proceedings of the Institution of Mechanical Engineers, Part J: Journal of Engineering Tribology*, 2007, *221* (3): 175-181.

[71] J. M. Clark. The Organization of Collagen in Cryofractured Rabbit Articular Cartilage: A Scanning Electron Microscopic Study [J]. *Journal of Orthopaedic Research*, 1985, *3* (1): 17-29.

[72] J. M. Clark. Variation of Collagen Fiber Alignment in a Joint Surface: A Scanning Electron Microscope Study of the Tibial Plateau in Dog, Rabbit, and Man [J]. *Journal of Orthopaedic Research*, 1991, *9* (2): 246-257.

[73] J. M. Clark & E. Rudd. Cell Patterns in the Surface of Rabbit Articular Cartilage Revealed by the Backscatter Mode of Scanning Electron Microscopy [J]. *Journal of Orthopaedic Research*, 1991, *9* (2): 275-283.

[74] J. M. Coletti Jr., W. H. Akeson & S. L. Woo. A Comparison of the Physical Behavior of Normal Articular Cartilage and the Arthroplasty Surface [J]. *Journal of Bone and Joint Surgery—Series A*, 1972, *54* (1): 147-160.

[75] J. R. Foy, P. F. W. Iii, G. L. Powell, K. Ishihara, N. Nakabayashi & M. LaBerge. Effect of Phospholipidic Boundary Lubrication in Rigid and Compliant Hemiarthroplasty Models [J]. *Proceedings of the Institution of Mechanical Engineers, Part H: Journal of Engineering in Medicine*, 1999, *213* (1): 5-18.

[76] J. R. Parsons & J. Black. The Viscoelastic Shear Behavior of Normal Rabbit Articular Cartilage [J]. *Journal of Biomechanics*, 1977, *10* (1): 21-29.

[77] J. R. Parsons & J. Black. Mechanical Behavior of Articular Cartilage: Quantitative Changes with Alteration of Ionic Environment [J]. *Journal of Biomechanics*, 1979, *12* (10): 765-773.

[78] J. S. Jurvelin, M. D. Buschmann & E. B. Hunziker. Optical and Mechanical Determination of Poisson's Ratio of Adult Bovine Humeral Articular Cartilage [J]. *Journal of Biomechanics*, 1997, *30* (3): 235-241.

[79] J. S. Rovick, J. D. Reuben, R. J. Schrager & P. S. Walker. Relation between Knee Motion and Ligament Length Patterns [J]. *Clinical Biomechanics*, 1991, *6* (4): 213-220.

[80] K. A. Athanasiou, A. Agarwal, A. Muffoletto, F. J. Dzida, G. Constantinides & M. Clem. Biomechanical Properties of Hip Cartilage in Experimental Animal Models [J]. *Clinical Orthopaedics and Related Research*, 1995 (316): 254-266.

[81] K. A. Athanasiou, M. P. Rosenwasser, J. A. Buckwalter, T. I. Malinin & V. C. Mow. Interspecies Comparisons of in Situ Intrinsic Mechanical Properties of Distal Femoral Cartilage [J]. *Journal of Orthopaedic Research*, 1991, *9* (3): 330-340.

[82] K. de Groot. Clinical Applications of Calcium Phosphate Biomaterials: A Review [J]. *Ceramics International*, 1993, *19* (5): 363-366.

[83] K. Friedrich, J. Karger-Kocsis, T. Sugioka & M. Yoshida. On the Sliding Wear Performance of Polyethernitrile Composites [J]. *Wear*, 1992, *158* (1-2): 157-170.

[84] K. O. Kjellsen & H. M. Jennings. Observations of Microcracking in Cement Paste upon Drying and Rewetting by Environmental Scanning Electron Microscopy [J]. *Advanced Cement Based Materials*, 1996, *3* (1): 14-19.

[85] L. A. Setton, W. Zhu & V. C. Mow. The Biphasic Poroviscoelastic Behavior of Articular Cartilage: Role of the Surface Zone in Governing the Compressive Behavior [J]. *Journal of Biomechanics*, 1993, *26* (4-5): 581-592.

[86] L. Ali & M. A. Barrufet. Study of Pore Structure Modification Using Environmental Scanning Electron Microscopy [J]. *Journal of Petroleum Science and Engineering*, 1995, *12* (4): 323-338.

[87] L. C. Clarke. The Microevaluation of Articular Surface Contours [J]. *Annals of Biomedical Engineering*, 1972, *1* (1): 31-43.

[88] L. G. M. De Bont, G. Boering, P. Havinga & R. S. B. Liem. Spatial Arrangement of Collagen Fibrils in the Articular Cartilage of the Mandibular Condyle: A Light Microscopic and Scanning Electron Microscopic Study [J]. *Journal of Oral and Maxillofacial Surgery*, 1984, *42*(5): 306-313.

[89] L. P. Zichner & H. G. Willert. Comparison of Alumina-Polyethylene and Metal-Polyethylene in Clinical Trials [J]. *Clinical Orthopaedics and Related Research*, 1992 (282): 86-94.

[90] L. Sokoloff. Elasticity of Articular Cartilage: Effect of Ions and Viscous Solutions [J]. *Science*, 1963, *141* (3585): 1055-1057.

[91] L. Sokoloff. Elasticity of Aging Cartilage [J]. *Federation Proceedings*, 1966, *25*(3): 1089-1095.

[92] M. A. Soltz & G. A. Ateshian. Experimental Verification and Theoretical Prediction of Cartilage Interstitial Fluid Pressurization at an Impermeable Contact Interface in Confined Compression [J]. *Journal of Biomechanics*, 1998, *31* (10): 927-934.

[93] M. A. Soltz & G. A. Ateshian. A Conewise Linear Elasticity Mixture Model for the Analysis of Tension-Compression Nonlinearity in Articular Cartilage [J]. *Journal of Biomechanical Engineering*, 2000, *122* (6): 576-586.

[94] M. E. Freeman, M. J. Furey, B. J. Love & J. M. Hampton. Friction, Wear, and Lubrication of Hydrogels as Synthetic Articular Cartilage [J]. *Wear*, 2000, *241* (2): 129-135.

[95] M. Hiroshi Naka, M. Hasuo, Y. Fuwa & K. Ikeuchi. Correlation Between Friction of Articular Cartilage and Reflectance Intensity From Superficial Images [J]. *Tribology International*, 2007, *40* (2 SPEC. ISS.): 200-207.

[96] M. I. Froimson, A. Ratcliffe, T. R. Gardner & V.C. Mow. Differences in Patellofemoral Joint Cartilage Material Properties and Their Significance to the Etiology of Cartilage Surface Fibrillation [J]. *Osteoarthritis and Cartilage*, 1997, *5* (6): 377-386.

[97] M. Kobayashi & M. Oka. The Lubricative Function of Artificial Joint Material Surfaces by Confocal Laser Scanning Microscopy: Comparison with Natural Synovial Joint Surface [J]. *Bio-Medical Materials and Engineering*, 2003, *13* (4): 429-437.

[98] M. Kobayashi, J. Toguchida & M. Oka. Preliminary Study of Polyvinyl Alcohol-Hydrogel (Pva-H) Artificial Meniscus [J]. *Biomaterials*, 2003, *24* (4): 639-647.

[99] M. Kobayashi, J. Toguchida & M. Oka. Study on the Lubrication Mechanism of Natural Joints by Confocal Laser Scanning Microscopy [J]. *Journal of Biomedical Materials Research*, 2001, *55* (4): 645-651.

[100] M. M. Lakouraj, M. Tajbakhsh & M. Mokhtary. Synthesis and Swelling Characterization of Cross-Linked Pvp/Pva Hydrogels [J]. *Iranian Polymer Journal (English Edition)*, 2005, *14* (12): 1022-1030.

[101] M. Okazaki, T. Hamada, H. Fujii, A. Mizobe & S. Matsuzawa. Development of Poly (Vinyl Alcohol) Hydrogel for Waste Water Cleaning. I. Study of Poly (Vinyl Alcohol) Gel as a Carrier for Immobilizing Microorganisms [J]. *Journal of Applied Polymer Science*, 1995, *58* (12): 2235-2241.

[102] M. Radice, P. Brun, R. Cortivo, R. Scapinelli, C. Battaliard & G. Abatangelo. Hyaluronan-Based Biopolymers as Delivery Vehicles for Bone-Marrow-Derived Mesenchymal Progenitors [J]. *Journal of Biomedical Materials Research*, 2000, *50* (2): 101-109.

[103] M. Ungethum & H. Stallforth. Systematy of Artificial Knee Joints Considering Constructional Characteristics of the Natural Knee Joint [J]. *Archiv für Orthopädische und Unfall-Chirurgie*, 1977, *89* (2): 227-237.

[104] M. Wong, M. Ponticiello, V. Kovanen & J. S. Jurvelin. Volumetric Changes of Articular Cartilage During Stress Relaxation in Unconfined Compression [J]. *Journal of Biomechanics*, 2000, *33* (9): 1049-1054.

[105] P. G. Bullough, P. S. Yawitz, L. Tafra & A. L. Boskey. Topographical Variations in the Morphology and Biochemistry of Adult Canine Tibial Plateau Articular Cartilage [J]. *Journal of Orthopaedic Research*, 1985, *3* (1): 1-16.

[106] P. G. Laing, A. B. Ferguson Jr. & E. S. Hodge. Tissue Reaction in Rabbit Muscle Exposed to Metallic Implants [J]. *Journal of Biomedical Materials Research*, 1967, *1* (1): 135-149.

[107] P. S. Walker, H. H. Hsieh. Conformity in Condylar Replacement Knee Prostheses [J]. *Journal of Bone and Joint Surgery—Series B*, 1977, *59* (2): 222-228.

[108] P. Tengvall, I. Lundstrom, C. Freij-Larsson, M. Kober & B. Wesslen. Ellipsometric Studies of Antisera Binding onto Medical Polyurethanes Immersed in Human Plasma in Vitro [J]. *Journal of Materials Science: Materials in Medicine*, 1993, *4* (3): 305-310.

[109] R. A. Brand. Joint Contact Stress: A Reasonable Surrogate for Biological

Processes? [J]. *The Iowa Orthopaedic Journal*, 2005(25): 82-94.

[110] R. Bader, E. Steinhauser, G. Willmann & R. Gradinger. Limitations of Artificial Hip Joint Mobility due to Wear and Ceramic Cup Design [J]. *Key Engineering Materials*, 2001 (192-195): 549-552.

[111] R. Crockett, S. Roos, P. Rossbach, C. Dora, W. Born & H. Troxler. Imaging of the Surface of Human and Bovine Articular Cartilage with Esem and AFM [J]. *Tribology Letters*, 2005, *19* (4): 311-317.

[112] R. D. Altman, J. Tenenbaum & L. Latta. Biomechanical and Biochemical Properties of Dog Cartilage in Experimentally Induced Osteoarthritis [J]. *Annals of the Rheumatic Diseases*, 1984, *43* (1): 83-90.

[113] R. D. Altman, M. C. Hochberg, R. W. Moskowitz & T. J. Schnitzer. Recommendations for the Medical Management of Osteoarthritis of the Hip and Knee: 2000 Update [J]. *Arthritis and Rheumatism*, 2000, *43* (9): 1905-1915.

[114] R. D. Komistek, D. A. Dennis, J. A. Mabe & S. A. Walker. An *in Vivo* Determination of Patellofemoral Contact Positions [J]. *Clinical Biomechanics*, 2000, *15* (1): 29-36.

[115] R. Ehrlich. An Alternative Method for Computing Contact Angle from the Dimensions of a Small Sessile Drop [J]. *Journal of Colloid and Interface Science*, 1967, *28* (1): 5-8.

[116] R. J. Covert, R. D. Ott & D. N. Ku. Friction Characteristics of a Potential Articular Cartilage Biomaterial [J]. *Wear*, 2003, *255* (7-12): 1064-1068.

[117] R. L. Buly, M. H. Huo, E. Salvati, W. Brien & M. Bansal. Titanium Wear Debris in Failed Cemented Total Hip Arthroplasty: An Analysis of 71 Cases [J]. *Journal of Arthroplasty*, 1992, *7* (3): 315-323.

[118] R. L. Spilker, J. K. Suh, M. E. Vermilyea & T. A. Maxian. *Biomechanics of Diarthrodial Joints* [M]. Berlin: Springer-Verlag, 1990

[119] R. M. Schinagl, D. Gurskis, A. C. Chen & R. L. Sah. Depth-Dependent Confined Compression Modulus of Full-Thickness Bovine Articular Cartilage [J]. *Journal of Orthopaedic Research*, 1997, *15* (4): 499-506.

[120] R. S. Burnett, R. B. Bourne. Indications for Patellar Resurfacing in Total Knee Arthroplasty [J]. *The Journal of Bone and Joint Surgery*, 2003, *85* (4): 728-745.

[121] R. S. Sayles, T. R. Thomas & J. Anderson. Measurement of the Surface

Microgeometry of Articular Cartilage [J]. *Journal of Biomechanics*, 1979, *12* (4): 257-267.

[122] R. T. Bothe, L. E. Beaton & H. A. Davenport. Reaction of Bone to Multiple Metallic Implants [J]. *Surg Gynecol Obstet*, 1940 (71): 598-602.

[123] R. W. Forsey, J. Fisher, J. Thompson, M. H. Stone, C. Bell & E. Ingham. The Effect of Hyaluronic Acid and Phospholipid Based Lubricants on Friction Within a Human Cartilage Damage Model [J]. *Biomaterials*, 2006, *27* (26): 4581-4590.

[124] R. Y. Hori & L. F. Mockros. Indentation Tests of Human Articular Cartilage [J]. *Journal of Biomechanics*, 1976, *9* (4): 259-268.

[125] S. Akizuki, V. C. Mow & F. Muller. Tensile Properties of Human Knee Joint Cartilage: I. Influence of Ionic Conditions, Weight Bearing, and Fibrillation on the Tensile Modulus [J]. *Journal of Orthopaedic Research*, 1986, *4* (4): 379-392.

[126] S. Byers, A. J. Moore, R. W. Byard & N. L. Fazzalari. Quantitative Histomorphometric Analysis of the Human Growth Plate from Birth to Adolescence [J]. *Bone*, 2000, *27* (4): 495-501.

[127] S. Graindorge, W. Ferrandez, E. Ingham, Z. Jin, P. Twigg & J. Fisher. The Role of the Surface Amorphous Layer of Articular Cartilage in Joint Lubrication [J]. *Proceedings of the Institution of Mechanical Engineers, Part H: Journal of Engineering in Medicine*, 2006, *220* (5): 597-607.

[128] S. Graindorge, W. Ferrandez, Z. Jin, E. Ingham & J. Fisher. The Natural Synovial Joint: A Finite Element Investigation of Biphasic Surface Amorphous Layer Lubrication under Dynamic Loading Conditions [J]. *Proceedings of the Institution of Mechanical Engineers, Part J: Journal of Engineering Tribology*, 2006, *220* (8): 671-681.

[129] S. H. Hyon, W. I. Cha & Y. Ikada. Preparation of Transparent Poly(Vinyl Alcohol) Hydrogel [J]. *Polymer Bulletin*, 1989, *22* (2): 119-122.

[130] S. Kobayashi, S. Yonekubo & Y. Kurogouchi. Cryoscanning Electron Microscopy of Loaded Articular Cartilage with Special Reference to the Surface Amorphous Layer [J]. *Journal of Anatomy*, 1996, *188* (2): 311-322.

[131] S. Kobayashi, S. Yonekubo & Y. Kurogouchi. Cryoscanning Electron Microscopic Study of the Surface Amorphous Layer of Articular Cartilage [J]. *Journal of Anatomy*, 1995, *187* (2): 429-444.

[132]S. L. Y. Woo, B R. Simon, S. C. Kuei & W. H. Akeson. Quasi-Linear Viscoelastic Properties of Normal Articular Cartilage [J]. *Journal of Biomechanical Engineering*, 1980, *102* (2): 85-90.

[133] S. M. Elmore, L. Sokoloff, G. Norris & P. Carmeci. Nature of "Imperfect" Elasticity of Articular Cartilage [J]. *J. Appl Physiol*, 1963, *18* (2): 393-396.

[134] S. S. Pawaskar, Z. M. Jin & J. Fisher. Modelling of Fluid Support inside Articular Cartilage During Sliding [J]. *Proceedings of the Institution of Mechanical Engineers, Part J: Journal of Engineering Tribology*, 2007, *221* (3): 165-174.

[135] S. W. Han & T. A. Blanchet. Experimental Evaluation of a Steady-State Model for the Wear of Particle-Filled Polymer Composite Materials [J]. *Journal of Tribology*, 1997, *119* (4): 694-699.

[136] T. A. Mahmood, V. P. Shastri, C. A. V. Blitterswijk, R. Langer & J. Riesle. Tissue Engineering of Bovine Articular Cartilage Within Porous Poly (Ether Ester) Copolymer Scaffolds with Different Structures [J]. *Tissue Engineering*, 2005, *11* (7-8): 1244-1253.

[137] T. Hardingham & M. Bayliss. Proteoglycans of Articular Cartilage: Changes in Aging and in Joint Disease [J]. *Seminars in Arthritis and Rheumatism*, 1991, *20* (3 SUPPL.1): 12-33.

[138] T. Hirai, H. Maruyama, T. Suzuki & S. Hayashi. Shape Memorizing Properties of a Hydrogel of Poly (Vinyl Alcohol) [J]. *Journal of Applied Polymer Science*, 1992 (45): 1849-1855.

[139] T. M. Guess & L. P. Maletsky. Computational Modelling of a Total Knee Prosthetic Loaded in a Dynamic Knee Simulator [J]. *Medical Engineering and Physics*, 2005, *27* (5): 357-367.

[140] V. Banchet, V. Fridrici, J. C. Abry & P. Kapsa. Wear and Friction Characterization of Materials for Hip Prosthesis [J]. *Wear*, 2007, *263* (7): 1066-1071.

[141] V. C. Mow & R. Huiskes. *Basic Orthopaedic Biomechanics & Mechano-Biology* [M]. Philadelphia: Lippincott Williams & Wilkins, 2004

[142] V. C. Mow & W. M. Lai. Mechanics of Animal Joints [J]. *Annual Review of Fluid Mechanics*, 1979 (11): 247-288.

[143] V. C. Mow & W. M. Lai. Recent Developments in Synovial Joint Biomechanics [J]. *SIAM Review*, 1980, *22* (3): 275-317.

[144] V. C. Mow, M. C. Gibbs, W. M. Lai, W. B. Zhu & K. A. Athanasiou. Biphasic Indentation of Articular Cartilage—Ii. A Numerical Algorithm and an Experimental Study [J]. *Journal of Biomechanics*, 1989, *22* (8-9): 853-861.

[145] V. C. Mow, S. C. Kuei, W. M. Lai & C. G. Armstrong. Biphasic Creep and Stress Relaxation of Articular Cartilage in Compression: Theory and Experiments [J]. *Journal of Biomechanical Engineering*, 1980, *102* (1): 73-84.

[146] V. C. Mow, W. M. Lai & M. H. Holmes. *Advanced Theoretical and Experimental Techniques in Cartilage Research* [M]. Nijmegen: Radboud University Press, 1982.

[147] Veeco Metrology Group. *Attaching Particles to AFM Cantilevers* [M]. New York: Veeco Metrology Group, 1996.

[148] Veeco Metrology Group. *Training Notebook* [M]. New York: Veeco Metrology Group, 1999.

[149] V. Saikko & T. Ahlroos, O. Calonius. A Three-Axis Knee Wear Simulator with Ball-on-Flat Contact [J]. *Wear*, 2001, *249* (3-4): 310-315.

[150] V. Wright & D. Dowson. Lubrication and Cartilage [J]. *Journal of Anatomy*, 1976, *121* (1): 107-118.

[151] W. A. Zisman. Relation of the Equilibrium Contact Angle to Liquid and Solid Constitution [J]. *Advances in Chemistry Series*, 1964 (43): 1-51.

[152] W. B. Bald & A.W. Robards. A Device for the Rapid Freezing of Biological Specimens Under Precisely Controlled and Reproducible Conditions [J]. *Journal of Microscopy*, 1978, *112* (1): 3-15.

[153] W. C. Hayes & A. J. Bodine. Flow-Independent Viscoelastic Properties of Articular Cartilage Matrix [J]. *Journal of Biomechanics*, 1978, *11* (8-9): 407-419.

[154] W. C. Hayes & L. F. Mockros. Viscoelastic Properties of Human Articular Cartilage [J]. *Journal of Applied Physiology*, 1971, *31* (4): 562-568.

[155] W. C. Hayes, L. M. Keer, G. Herrmann & L. F. Mockros. A Mathematical Analysis for Indentation Tests of Articular Cartilage [J]. *Journal of Biomechanics*, 1972, *5* (5): 541-551.

[156] W. C. Witzleb, J. Ziegler, F. Krummenauer, V. Neumeister & K. P. Guenther. Exposure to Chromium, Cobalt and Molybdenum from Metal-on-Metal Total Hip Replacement and Hip Resurfacing Arthroplasty [J]. *Acta Orthopaedica*, 2006, *77* (5): 697-705.

[157] W. I. Cha, S. H. Hyon, M. Oka & Y. Ikada. Mechanical and Wear Properties of Poly (Vinyl Alcohol) Hydrogels [J]. *Macromolecular Symposia*, 1996 (109): 115-126.

[158] W. M. Lai, J. S. Hou & V. C. Mow. A Triphasic Theory for the Swelling and Deformation Behaviors of Articular Cartilage [J]. *Journal of Biomechanical Engineering*, 1991, *113* (3): 245-258.

[159] W. T. Green Jr. Articular Cartilage Repair: Behavior of Rabbit Chondrocytes During Tissue Culture and Subsequent Allografting [J]. *Clinical Orthopaedics and Related Research*, 1977 (124): 237-250.

[160] W. Wilson, C. C. V. Donkelaar, B. V. Rietbergen & R. Huiskes. A Fibril-Reinforced Poroviscoelastic Swelling Model for Articular Cartilage [J]. *Journal of Biomechanics*, 2005, *38* (6): 1195-1204.

[161] X. L. Lu, D. D. N. Sun, X. E. Guo, F. H. Chen, W. M. Lai & V. C. Mow. Indentation Determined Mechanoelectrochemical Properties and Fixed Charge Density of Articular Cartilage [J]. *Annals of Biomedical Engineering*, 2004, *32* (3): 370-379.

[162] Y. Sawae, T. Murakami & J. Chen. Effect of Synovia Constituents on Friction and Wear of Ultra-High Molecular Weight Polyethylene Sliding Against Prosthetic Joint Materials [J]. *Wear*, 1998, *216* (2): 213-219.

[163] Y. S. Pan, D. S. Xiong & R. Y. Ma. A Study on the Friction Properties of Poly (Vinyl Alcohol) Hydrogel as Articular Cartilage against Titanium Alloy [J]. *Wear*, 2007, *262* (7-8): 1021-1025.